T0222210

# HISTOLOGY OF THE BLOOD

## NORMAL AND PATHOLOGICAL.

# HISTOLOGY OF THE BLOOD

## NORMAL AND PATHOLOGICAL

BY

## P. EHRLICH AND A. LAZARUS.

EDITED AND TRANSLATED

BY

## W. MYERS, M.A., M.B., B.Sc.
JOHN LUCAS WALKER STUDENT OF PATHOLOGY.

WITH A PREFACE

BY

## G. SIMS WOODHEAD, M.D.
PROFESSOR OF PATHOLOGY IN THE UNIVERSITY OF CAMBRIDGE.

CAMBRIDGE:
AT THE UNIVERSITY PRESS.

1900

# CAMBRIDGE
## UNIVERSITY PRESS

University Printing House, Cambridge CB2 8BS, United Kingdom

Cambridge University Press is part of the University of Cambridge.

It furthers the University's mission by disseminating knowledge in the pursuit of
education, learning and research at the highest international levels of excellence.

www.cambridge.org
Information on this title: www.cambridge.org/9781107450868

© Cambridge University Press 1900

First published 1900
First paperback edition 2014

A catalogue record for this publication is available from the British Library

ISBN 978-1-107-45086-8 Paperback

# PREFACE.

IN no department of Pathology has advance been so fitful and interrupted as in that dealing with blood changes in various forms of disease, though none now offers a field that promises such an abundant return for an equal expenditure of time and labour.

Observations of great importance were early made by Wharton Jones, Waller, and Hughes Bennett in this country, and by Virchow and Max Schultze in Germany. Not, however, until the decade ending in 1890 was it realised what a large amount of new work on the corpuscular elements of the blood had been done by Hayem, and by Ehrlich and his pupils. As successive papers were published, especially from German laboratories, it became evident that the systematic study of the blood by various new methods was resulting in the acquisition of a large number of facts bearing on the pathology of the blood; though it was still difficult to localise many of the normal hæmatogenetic processes. The production of the various cells under pathological conditions, where so many new factors are introduced, must necessarily be enshrouded in even greater obscurity and could only be accurately determined by patient investigation, a careful arrangement and study of facts, and cautious deduction from accumulated and classified observations.

The pathology of the blood, especially of the corpuscular elements, though one of the most interesting, is certainly one of the most confusing, of all departments of pathology, and to those who have not given almost undivided attention to this subject it is extremely difficult to obtain a comprehensive and accurate view of the blood in disease. It is for this reason that we welcome the present work in its English garb. Professor Ehrlich by his careful and extended observations on the blood has qualified himself to give a bird's-eye view of the subject, such as few if any are capable of offering; and his book now so well translated by Mr Myers must remain one of the classical works on blood in disease and on blood diseases, and in introducing it to English readers Mr Myers makes an important contribution to the accurate study of hæmal pathology in this country.

Comparatively few amongst us are able to make a cytological examination of the blood, whilst fewer still are competent to interpret the results of such an examination. How many of our physicians are in a position to distinguish between a myelogenic leukocythæmia and a lymphatic leukæmia? How many of us could draw correct inferences from the fact that in typhoid fever there may not only be no increase in the number of certain of the white cells of the blood, but an actual leukopenia? How many appreciated the diagnostic value of the difference in the cellular elements in the blood in cases of scarlet fever and of measles, and how many have anything more than a general idea as to the significance of a hypoleucocytosis or a hyperleucocytosis in a case of acute pneumonia, or as to the relations of cells of different forms and the percentage quantity of hæmoglobin found in the various types of anæmia ?

One of the most important points indicated in the following pages is that the cellular elements of the blood must be studied as a whole and not as isolated factors, as " it has always been shown that the character of a leukæmic condition is only settled by a concurrence of a large number of single symptoms of which each one is indispensable for the diagnosis, and which taken together are absolutely conclusive." Conditions of experiment can of course be carefully determined, so far, at any rate, as the introduction of substances from outside is concerned, but we must always bear in mind that it is impossible, except in very special cases of disease, to separate the action of the bone-marrow from the action of the lymphatic glands ; still, by careful observation and in special cases, especially when the various organs and parts may be examined after death, information may be gained even on this point. By means of experiment the production of leucocytosis by peptones, the action of micro-organisms on the bone-marrow, the influence of the products of decaying or degenerating epithelial or endothelioid cells, may all be studied in a more or less perfect form ; but, withal, it is only by a study of the numerous conditions under which alterations in the cellular elements take place in the blood that any accurate information can be obtained.

Hence for further knowledge of the "structure" and certain functions of the blood we must to a great extent rely upon clinical observation.

Some of the simpler problems have already been flooded with light by those who following in Ehrlich's footsteps have studied the blood in disease. But many of even greater importance might be cited from the work before us. With the abundant information, the well argued deductions and the carefully drawn up statement here placed before us it may be claimed that we are now in a position to make diagnoses that not long ago were quite beyond our reach, whilst a thorough training of our younger medical men in the methods of blood examination must result in the accumulation of new facts of prime importance both to the pathologist and to the physician.

Both teacher and investigator cannot but feel that they have now at command not only accurate results obtained by careful observation, but the foundation on which the superstructure has been built up—exquisite but simple methods of research. Ehrlich's methods may be (and have already been) somewhat modified as occasion requires, but the principles of fixation and staining here set forth must for long remain the methods to be utilised in future work. His differential staining, in which he utilised the special affinities that certain cells and parts of cells have for basic, acid and neutral stains, was simply a foreshadowing of his work on the affinity that certain cells and tissues have for specific drugs and toxins; the study of these special elective affinities now forms a very wide field of investigation in which numerous workers are already engaged in determining the position and nature of these seats of election for special proteid and other poisons.

The researches of Metschnikoff, of Kanthack and Hardy, of Muir, of Buchanan, and others, are supplementary and complementary to those carried on in the German School, but we may safely say that this work must be looked upon as influencing the study of blood more than any that has yet been published. It is only after a careful study of this book that any idea of the enormous amount of work that has been contributed to hæmatology by Ehrlich and his pupils, and the relatively important part that such a work must play in guiding and encouraging those who are interested in this fascinating subject, can be formed.

The translation appears to have been very carefully made, and the opportunity has been seized to add notes on certain points that have a special bearing on Ehrlich's work, or that have been brought into prominence since the time that the original work was produced. This renders the English edition in certain respects superior even to the original.

G. SIMS WOODHEAD.

# NOTE BY THE TRANSLATOR.

THIS translation of the first part of *Die Anæmie,*
*Nothnagel's Specielle Pathologie und Therapie,*
vol. VIII. was carried out under the personal guidance
of Professor Ehrlich. Several alterations and additions
have been made in the present edition. To my friend
Dr Cobbett I owe a debt of gratitude for his kind help
in the revision of the proof-sheets.

W. M.

# CONTENTS.

# INTRODUCTION.

## DEFINITION OF ANÆMIA. CLINICAL METHODS OF INVESTIGATION OF THE BLOOD.

In practical medicine the term "anæmia" has not quite the restricted sense that scientific investigation gives it. The former regards certain striking symptoms as characteristic of the anæmic condition; pallor of the skin, a diminution of the normal redness of the mucous membranes of the eyes, lips, mouth, and pharynx. From the presence of these phenomena anæmia is diagnosed, and according to their greater or less intensity, conclusions are also drawn as to the degree of the poverty of the blood.

It is evident from the first that a definition based on such a frequent and elementary chain of symptoms will bring into line much that is unconnected, and will perhaps omit what it should logically include. Indeed a number of obscurities and contradictions is to be ascribed to this circumstance.

The first task therefore of a scientific treatment of the anæmic condition is carefully to define its extent. For this purpose the symptoms above mentioned are little suited, however great, in their proper place, their practical importance may be.

Etymologically the word "anæmia" signifies a

1

want of the normal quantity of blood. This may be "general" and affect the whole organism; or "local" and limited to a particular region or a single organ. The local anæmias we can at once exclude from our consideration.

*A priori*, the amount of blood may be subnormal in two senses, quantitative and qualitative. We may have a diminution of the amount of blood—"Oligæmia." Deterioration of the quality of the blood may be quite independent of the amount of blood, and must primarily express itself in a diminution of the physiologically important constituents. Hence we distinguish the following chief types of alteration of the blood; (1) diminution of the amount of Hæmoglobin (Oligochromæmia), and (2) diminution of the number of red blood corpuscles (Oligocythæmia).

We regard as anæmic all conditions of the blood where a diminution of the amount of hæmoglobin can be recognised; in by far the greater number of cases, if not in all, Oligæmia and Oligocythæmia to a greater or less extent occur simultaneously.

The most important methods of clinical hæmatology bear directly or indirectly on the recognition of these conditions.

There is at present no method of ESTIMATION OF THE TOTAL QUANTITY OF THE BLOOD which can be used clinically. We rely to a certain extent on the observation of the already mentioned symptoms of redness or pallor of the skin and mucous membranes. To a large degree these depend upon the composition of the blood, and not upon the fulness of the peripheral vessels. If we take the latter as a measure of the total amount of blood, isolated vessels, visible to the naked eye, *e.g.* those of the sclerotic, may be observed. Most suitable is the ophthalmoscopic examination of the width of the vessels at the back of the eye. Ræhlmann has shewn that in 60 % of the cases of chronic anæmia, in which the skin and mucous membranes are very white, there is hyperæmia of the retina—which is evidence that in such cases the circulating blood is pale in colour, but certainly not less in quantity than normally. The condition of the pulse is an important indication of diminution of the quantity of the blood, though only when it is marked. It presents a peculiar smallness and feebleness in all cases of severe oligæmia.

The bleeding from fresh skin punctures gives a further criterion of the quantity of blood, within certain limits, but is modified by changes in the coagulability of the blood. Anyone who has made frequent blood examinations will have observed that in this respect extraordinary variations occur. In some cases scarcely a drop of blood can be obtained, while in others the blood flows freely. One will not err in assuming in the former case a diminution of the quantity of the blood.

The fulness of the peripheral vessels however is a sign of only relative value, for the amount of blood in the internal organs may be very different. The problem, how to estimate exactly, if possible mathematically, the quantity of blood in the body has always been recognised as important, and its solution would constitute a real advance. The methods which have so far been proposed for clinical purposes originate from Tarchanoff. He suggested that one may estimate the quantity of blood by comparing the numbers of the red blood corpuscles before and after copious sweating. Apart from various theoretical considerations this method is far too clumsy for practical purposes.

Quincke has endeavoured to calculate the amount of blood in cases of blood transfusion for therapeutic purposes. From the number of red blood corpuscles of the patient before and after blood transfusion, the amount of blood transfused and the number of corpuscles it contains, by a simple mathematical formula the quantity of the blood of the patient can be estimated. But this method is only practicable in special cases and is open to several theoretical errors. First, it depends upon the relative number of red blood corpuscles in the blood; inasmuch as the transfusion of normal blood into normal blood, for example, would produce no alteration in the count. This consideration is enough to shew that this proceeding can only be used in special cases. It has indeed been found that an increase of the red corpuscles per cubic millimetre occurs in persons with a very small number of red corpuscles, who have been injected with normal blood. But it is very hazardous to try to estimate therefrom the volume of the preexisting blood, since the act of transfusion undoubtedly is immediately followed by compensatory currents and alterations in the distribution of the blood.

No property of the blood has been so exactly and frequently tested as the NUMBER OF RED CORPUSCLES PER CUBIC MILLIMETRE OF BLOOD. The convenience of the counting apparatus, and the apparently absolute measure of the result have ensured for the methods of enumeration an early clinical application.

At the present time the instruments of Thoma-Zeiss or others similarly constructed are generally used; and we may assume that the principle on which they depend and the methods of their use are known. A number of fluids are used to dilute the blood, which on the whole fulfil the requirements of preserving the form and colour of the red corpuscles, of preventing their fusing together, and of allowing them to settle rapidly. Of the better known solutions we will here mention Pacini's and Hayem's fluids.

| | | |
|---|---|---|
| Pacini's solution. | Hydrarg. bichlor. | 2·0 |
| | Natr. chlor. | 4·0 |
| | Glycerin | 26·0 |
| | Aquæ destillat. | 226·0 |
| Hayem's solution. | Hydrarg. bichlor. | 0·5 |
| | Natr. sulph. | 5·0 |
| | Natr. chlor. | 1·0 |
| | Aquæ destillat. | 200·0 |

For counting the white blood corpuscles the same instrument is generally used, but the blood is diluted 10 times instead of 100 times. It is advantageous to use a diluting fluid which destroys the red blood corpuscles, but which brings out the nuclei of the white corpuscles, so that the latter are more easily recognised. For this purpose the solution recommended by Thoma is the best—namely a half per cent. solution of acetic acid, to which a trace of methyl violet has been added[1].

The results of these methods of enumeration are sufficiently exact, as they have, according to the frequently confirmed observations of R. Thoma and I. F. Lyon, only a small error. In a count of 200 cells it is five per cent., of 1250 two per cent., of 5000 one, and of 20,000 one-half per cent.

There are certain factors in the practical application of these methods, which in other directions influence the result unfavourably.

[1] For the estimation of the numbers of white corpuscles, relatively to the red, and of the different kinds relatively to each other, see the section on the morphology.

It has been found by Cohnstein and Zuntz and others that the blood in the large vessels has a constant composition, but that in the small vessels and capillaries the formed elements may vary considerably in number, though the blood is in other respects normal. Thus, for example, in a one-sided paralytic, the capillary blood is different on the two sides; and congestion, cold, and so forth raise the number of red blood corpuscles. Hence, for purposes of enumeration, the rule is to take blood only from those parts of the body which are free from accidental variation; to avoid all influences such as energetic rubbing or scrubbing, etc., which alter the circulation in the capillaries; to undertake the examination at such times when the number of red blood corpuscles is not influenced by the taking of food or medicine.

It is usual to take the blood from the tip of the finger, and only in exceptional cases, *e.g.* in œdema of the finger, are other places chosen, such as the lobule of the ear, or (in the case of children) the big toe. For the puncture pointed needles or specially constructed instruments, open or shielded lancets, are unnecessary: we recommend a fine steel pen, of which one nib has been broken off. It is easily disinfected by heating to redness, and produces not a puncture but what is more useful, a cut, from which blood freely flows without any great pressure.

The literature dealing with the numbers of the red corpuscles in health, is so large as to be quite unsurveyable. According to the new and complete compilation of Reinert and v. Limbeck, the following figures (calculated roundly for mm.³) may be taken as physiological:

## Men.

| Maximum | Minimum | Average |
|---------|---------|---------|
| 7,000,000 | 4,000,000 | 5,000,000 |

## Women.

| Maximum | Minimum | Average |
|---------|---------|---------|
| 5,250,000 | 4,500,000 | 4,500,000 |

This difference between the sexes first makes its appearance at the time of puberty of the female. Up to the commencement of menstruation the number of corpuscles in the female is in fact slightly higher than in the male (Stierlin). Apart from this, the time of life seems to cause a difference in the number of red corpuscles only in so far that in the newly-born, polycythæmia (up to $8\frac{1}{2}$ millions during the first days of life) is observed (E. Schiff). After the first occasion on which food is taken a decrease can be observed, and gradually (though by stages) the normal figure is reached in from 10–14 days. On the other hand the oligocythæmia here and there observed in old age, according to Schmaltz, is not constant, and therefore cannot be regarded as a peculiarity of senility, but must be caused by subsidiary processes of various kinds which come into play at this stage of life.

The influence which the taking of food exercises on the number of the red blood corpuscles is to be ascribed to the taking in of water, and is so insignificant, that the variations, in part at least, fall within the errors of the methods of enumeration.

Other physiological factors : menstruation (that is, the single occurrence), pregnancy, lactation, do not alter the number of blood corpuscles to any appreciable extent. The numbers do not differ in arterial and venous blood.

All these physiological variations in the number of the blood corpuscles, are dependent, according to Cohnstein and Zuntz, on vasomotor influences. Stimuli, which narrow the peripheral vessels, locally diminish the number of red blood corpuscles; excitation of the vasodilators brings about the opposite effect. Hence it follows, that the normal variations of the number contained in a unit of space are merely the expressions of an altered distribution of the red elements within the circulation, and are quite independent of the reproduction and decay of the cells.

Climatic conditions apparently exercise a great influence over the number of corpuscles. This fact is important for physiology, pathology, and therapeutics, and has come to the front especially in the last few years, since Viault's researches in the heights of the Corderillas. As his researches, as well as those of Mercier, Egger, Wolff, Kœppe, v. Jaruntowski and Schrœder, Miescher, Kündig and others, shew, the number of red blood corpuscles in a healthy man, with the normal average of 5,000,000 per mm.³, begins to rise immediately after reaching a height considerably above the sealevel. With a rise proceeding by stages, a new average figure is reached in 10 to 14 days, considerably larger than the old one, and indeed the greater the difference in level between the former and the latter places, the greater is the difference in this figure. Healthy persons born and bred at these heights have an average of red corpuscles which is considerably above the mean; and which indeed as a rule is somewhat greater than in those who are acclimatised or only temporarily living at these elevations.

The following small table gives an idea of the degree

to which the number of blood corpuscles may vary at higher altitudes from the average of five millions.

| Author | Locality | Height above sea-level | Increase of |
|---|---|---|---|
| v. Jaruntowski | Görbersdorf | 561 metres | 800,000 |
| Wolff and Kœppe | Reiboldsgrün | 700 ,, | 1,000,000 |
| Egger ... ... | Arosa ... | 1800 ,, | 2,000,000 |
| Viault ... ... | Corderillas | 4392 ,, | 3,000,000 |

Exactly the opposite process is to be observed when a person accustomed to a high altitude reaches a lower one. Under these conditions the correspondingly lower physiological average is produced. These interesting processes have given rise to various interpretations and hypotheses. On the one hand, the diminished oxygen tension in the upper air was regarded as the immediate cause of the increase of red blood corpuscles. Miescher, particularly, has described the want of oxygen as a specific stimulus to the production of erythrocytes. Apart from the physiological improbability of such a rapid and comprehensive fresh production, one must further dissent from this interpretation, since the histological appearance of the blood gives it no support. Kœppe, who has specially directed part of his researches to the morphological phenomena produced during acclimatisation to high altitudes, has shewn, that in the increase of the number of red corpuscles two mutually independent and distinct processes are to be distinguished. He observed that, although the number of red corpuscles was raised so soon as a few hours after arrival at Reiboldsgrün, numerous poikilocytes and microcytes make their appearance at the same time. The initial increase is therefore to be explained by budding and division of the red corpuscles already present in the circulating blood. Kœppe sees in this process, borrowing Ehrlich's conception of poikilocytosis, a physiological adaptation to the lower atmospheric pressure, and the resulting greater difficulty of oxygen absorption. The impediment to the function of the hæmoglobin is to a certain extent compensated, since the stock of hæmoglobin possesses a larger surface, and so is capable of increased respiration. So also the remarkable fact may be readily understood that the sudden rise of the number of corpuscles is not at first accompanied by a rise of the quantity of hæmoglobin, or of the total volume of the red blood corpuscles. These values are first increased when the second process, an increased fresh production of normal red discs, takes place, which naturally requires for its developement a longer time. The poikilocytes and microcytes then vanish, according to the extent of the reproduction; and finally a blood is formed, which is characterised by an increased number of red corpuscles, and a corresponding rise in the quantity of hæmoglobin, and in the percentage volume of the corpuscles.

Other authors infer a relative and not an absolute increase in the number of red corpuscles. E. Grawitz, for example, has expressed the opinion that the raised count of corpuscles may be explained chiefly by increased concentration of the blood, due to the greater loss of water from the body at these altitudes. The blood of laboratory animals which Grawitz allowed to live in correspondingly rarefied air underwent similar changes. Von Limbeck, as well as Schumburg and Zuntz, object to this explanation on the ground, that if loss of water caused such considerable elevations in the number, we should observe a corresponding diminution in the body weight, which is by no means the case.

Schumburg and Zuntz also regard the increase of red blood corpuscles in the higher mountains as relative only, but explain it by an altered distribution of the corpuscular elements within the vascular system. In their earlier work Cohnstein and Zuntz had already established that the number of corpuscles in the capillary blood varies with the width of the vessels and the rate of flow in them. If one reflects how multifarious are the merely physiological influences at the bottom of which these two factors lie, one will not interpret alterations in the number of the red corpuscles without bearing them in mind. In residence at high altitudes various factors bring about alterations in the width of the vessels and in the circulation. Amongst these are the intenser light (Fülles), the lowering of temperature, increased muscular exertion, raised respiratory activity. Doubtless, therefore, without either production of microcytes or production *de novo*, the number of red corpuscles in capillary blood may undergo considerable variations.

The opposition, in which as mentioned above, the views of Grawitz, Zuntz, and Schumburg stand to those of the first mentioned authors, finds its solution in the fact that the causes of altered distribution of the blood, and of loss of water, play a large part in the sudden changes. The longer the sojourn however at these great elevations, the more insignificant they become (Viault).

We think therefore that from the material before us we may draw the conclusion, that after long residence in elevated districts the number of red blood corpuscles is absolutely raised. The therapeutic importance of this influence is obvious.

Besides high altitudes, the influence of the tropics

on the composition of the blood and especially on the number of corpuscles has also been tested. Eykmann as well as Glogner found no deviation from the normal, although the almost constant pallor of the European in the tropics points in that direction. Here also, changes in the distribution occurring without qualitative changes of the blood seem chiefly concerned.

---

The same reliance cannot be placed on inferences based on the results of the Thoma-Zeiss and similar counting methods for anæmic as for normal blood, in which generally speaking all the red cells are of the same size and contain the same amount of hæmoglobin. In the former the red corpuscles, as we shall shew later, differ considerably one from another. On the one hand forms poor in hæmoglobin, on the other very small forms occur, which by the wet method of counting cannot even be seen.

Apart even from these extreme forms, 1,000 red blood corpuscles of anæmic blood are not physiologically equivalent to the same number of normal blood corpuscles. Hence the necessity of closely correlating the result of the count of red blood corpuscles with the hæmoglobinometric and histological values. The first figure only, given apart from the latter, is often misleading, especially in pathological cases.

It is therefore occasionally desirable to supplement the data of the count by THE ESTIMATION OF THE SIZE OF THE RED BLOOD CORPUSCLES INDIVIDUALLY. This is effected by direct measurement with the ocular micrometer; and can be performed on wet (see below), as well as on dry preparations, though the latter in general are to be preferred on account of their far greater convenience.

Nevertheless the carrying out of this method requires particular care. One can easily see that in normal blood the red corpuscles appear smaller in the thicker than they do in the thinner layers of the dry preparation. We may explain this difference as follows. In the thick layers the red discs float in plasma before drying, whilst in the thinner parts they are fastened to the glass by a capillary layer. Desiccation occurs here nearly instantaneously, and starts from the periphery of the disc; so that an alteration in the shape or size is impossible. On the contrary the process of drying in the thicker portions proceeds more slowly, and is therefore accompanied by a shrinking of the discs.

Even in healthy persons small differences in the individual discs are shewn by this method. The physiological average of the diameter of the greater surface is, according to Laache, Hayem, Schumann and others, $8\cdot5\,\mu$ for men and women (max. $9\cdot0\,\mu$. min. $6\cdot5\,\mu$.) In anæmic blood the differences between the individual elements become greater, so that to obtain the average value, the maxima, minima, and mean of a large number of cells, chosen at random, are ascertained. But with a high degree of inequality of the discs this microscopical measurement loses all scientific value.

However valuable the knowledge of the absolute number may be for a judgment on the course of the illness, it gives us no information about the AMOUNT OF HÆMOGLOBIN IN THE BLOOD, which is the decisive measure of the degree of the anæmia. A number of clinical methods are in use for this estimation; first direct, such as the colorimetric estimation of the amount of hæmo-globin, secondly indirect, such as the determination of the specific gravity or of the volume of the red corpuscles, and perhaps also the estimation of the dry substance of the total blood.

Among the direct methods for hæmoglobin estimation, which aim at the measurement of the depth of colour of the blood, we wish first to mention one, which though it lays no claim to great clinical accuracy has often done us good service as a rapid indicator at the bed-side. A little blood is caught on a piece of linen or filter-paper, and allowed to distribute itself in a thin layer. In this manner one can recognise the difference between the colour of anæmic and of healthy blood more clearly than in the drop as it comes from the finger prick. After a few trials one can in this way draw conclusions as to the degree of the existing anæmia. Could this simple method which is so convenient, which can be carried out at the time of consultation, come more into vogue, it alone would con-tribute to the decline of the favourite stop-gap diagnosis, 'anæmia.' For neurasthenic patients also, who so often fancy themselves anæmic and in addition look so, a *demon-stratio ad oculos* such as this is often sufficient to persuade them of the contrary.

Of the instruments for measuring the depth of colour of the blood, the double pipette of Hoppe-Seyler is quite the most delicate. A solution of carbonic oxide hæmoglobin, accurately titrated, serves as the standard of comparison. The reliable preparation and conservation of the normal solution is however attended with such difficulties, that this method is not clinically available. In the last few years, Langemeister, a pupil of Kühne's, has invented a method for colorimetric purposes, also applicable to hæmoglobin estimations. The instrument depends on the principle, that from the thickness of the layer in which the solution to be tested has the same colour intensity as a normal solution, the amount of colour can be calculated. As a normal solution Langemeister uses a glycerine solution of methæmoglobin prepared from pig's blood. To our knowledge this method has not yet been applied clinically. Its introduction would be valuable, for in practice we must at present be content with methods that are less exact, in which coloured glass or a stable coloured solution serves as a measure for the depth of colour of the blood. There are a number of instruments of this kind, of which the "hæmometer" of Fleischl, and amongst others, the "hæmoglobinometer" of Gowers, distinguished by its low price, are specially used for clinical purposes. Both instruments give the percentage of the hæmoglobin of normal blood which the blood examined contains, and are sufficiently exact in their results for practical purposes and for relative values ; although errors up to 10 $\%$ and over occur with unpractised observers. (Cp. K. H. Mayer.) Quite recently Biernacki has raised the objection to the colorimetric methods of the quantitative estimation of hæmoglobin, that the depth of colour of the blood is dependent not only on the quantity of hæmoglobin but also on the colour of the plasma, and the greater or less amount of proteid in the blood. These errors are quite inconsiderable for the above-mentioned instruments, since here the blood is so highly diluted with water that the possible original differences are thereby reduced to zero.

Among the methods for indirect hæmoglobin estimation, that of calculation from the amount of iron in the blood appears to be quite exact, since hæmoglobin

possesses a constant quantity of iron of 0·42 per cent.
This calculation may be allowed in all cases for normal
blood, for here there is a really exact proportion between
the amounts of hæmoglobin and of iron. Recently A. Jolles
has described an apparatus for quantitative estimation
of the iron of the blood, called a "ferrometer;" which
renders possible an accurate valuation of the iron in small
amounts of blood. However for pathological cases this
method of hæmoglobin estimation from the iron present
is not to be recommended. For if one tests the blood of
an anæmic patient under the microscope for iron one finds
the iron reaction in numerous red blood corpuscles. This
means the presence of iron which is not a normal constituent of hæmoglobin. Other iron may be contained
in the morphological elements (including the white corpuscles) as a combination of proteid with iron, which is
not directly recognisable. It is further known that in
anæmias the amount of iron of all organs is greatly
raised (Quincke), apparently often the result of a raised
destruction of hæmoglobin ("waste iron," "spodogenous
iron"). In many cases too it should be borne in mind
that the administration of iron increases the amount of
iron in the blood and organs.

From these considerations we see how unreliable in
pathological cases is the calculation of the amount of
hæmoglobin from the amount of iron. We have been
particularly led to these observations by the work of
Biernacki, since the procedure of inferring the amount
of hæmoglobin from the amount of iron has led to really
remarkable conclusions. For example, amongst other
things, he found the iron in two cases of mild, and one
of severe chlorosis quite normal. He concludes that
chlorosis, and other anæmias, shew no diminution, but

even a relative increase of hæmoglobin: but that other proteids of the blood on the contrary are reduced. These difficult iron estimations stand out very sharply from the results of other authors and could only be accepted after the most careful confirmation. But the above analysis shews, that in any case the far-reaching conclusions which Biernacki has attached to his results are insecure. For these questions especially, complete estimations with the aid of the ferrometer of A. Jolles are to be desired.

Great importance has always been attached to the investigation of the SPECIFIC GRAVITY of the blood; since the density of the blood affords a measure of the number of corpuscles, and of their hæmoglobin equivalent. It is easy to collect observations, as in the last few years two methods have come into use which require only a small quantity of material, and do not appear to be too complicated for practical clinical purposes. One of these has been worked out by R. Schmaltz, in which small amounts of blood are exactly weighed in capillary glass tubes (the capillary pyknometric method). The other is A. Hammerschlag's, in which, by a variation of a principle which was first invented by Fano, that mixture of chloroform and benzol is ascertained in which the blood to be examined floats, *i.e.* which possesses exactly the specific gravity of the blood[1].

According to the researches of these authors and

---

[1] In Roy's method, mixtures of glycerine and water are used. By means of a curved pipette, the drop of blood is brought into the fluid, and its immediate motion observed. Lazarus Barlow has modified this method. He employs mixtures of gum and water, and instead of several tubes, one only; and into this the mixtures are introduced, those of higher specific gravity being naturally at the bottom. The alternate layers are coloured, and remain distinguishable for several hours.

numerous others who have used their own methods, the specific gravity of the total blood is physiologically 1058—1062, or on the average 1059 (1056 in women). The specific gravity of the serum amounts to 1029—1032 —on the average 1030. From which it at once follows that the red corpuscles must be the chief cause of the great weight of the blood. If their number diminishes, or their number remaining constant, they lose in hæmoglobin, or in volume, the specific gravity would be correspondingly lowered. We should therefore expect a low specific gravity in all anæmic conditions. Similarly with an increased number of corpuscles, and a high hæmoglobin equivalent, an increase in the density of the total blood makes its appearance.

Hammerschlag has found in a large number of experiments that the relation between the specific gravity and the amount of hæmoglobin is much closer than between the specific gravity and the number of corpuscles. The former in fact is so constant that it may be represented by a table.

| Sp. gravity | | | Quantity of Hæmoglobin (Fleischl's method) |
|---|---|---|---|
| 1033–1035 | ... | ... | 25–30 $^0/_0$ |
| 1035–1038 | ... | ... | 30–35 $^0/_0$ |
| 1038–1040 | ... | ... | 35–40 $^0/_0$ |
| 1040–1045 | ... | ... | 40–45 $^0/_0$ |
| 1045–1048 | ... | ... | 45–55 $^0/_0$ |
| 1048–1050 | ... | ... | 55–65 $^0/_0$ |
| 1050–1053 | ... | ... | 65–70 $^0/_0$ |
| 1053–1055 | ... | ... | 70–75 $^0/_0$ |
| 1055–1057 | ... | ... | 75–85 $^0/_0$ |
| 1057–1060 | ... | ... | 85–95 $^0/_0$ |

In a paper which has quite recently appeared Diabella has investigated these relations very thoroughly, and his results partly correct, and partly confirm those of Hammerschlag. Diabella found from his comparative estimations that differences of 10% hæmoglobin (Fleischl) correspond in general to differences of 4·46 per thousand in the specific gravity (Hammerschlag's method). Nevertheless with the same amount of hæmoglobin, differences up to 13·5 per thousand are to be observed; and these departures are greater the richer the blood in hæmoglobin. Regular differences exist between men and women; the latter have, with the same amount of hæmoglobin, a specific gravity lower by 2 to 2·5.

Should the parallelism between the number of red blood corpuscles and the amount of hæmoglobin be considerably disturbed, the influence of the stroma of the red discs on the specific gravity of the blood will then be recognisable. Diabella calculates, that with the same amount of hæmoglobin in two blood testings, the stroma may effect differences of 3—5 per thousand in the specific gravity.

Hence the estimation of the specific gravity is often sufficient for the determination of the relative amount of hæmoglobin of a blood. It is only in cases of nephritis and in circulatory disturbances, and in leukæmia, that the relations between specific gravity and quantity of hæmoglobin are too much masked by other influences.

The physiological variations which the specific gravity undergoes under the influence of the taking in and excretion of fluid do not exceed 0·003 (Schmaltz). From what has been said, it follows that all variations must correspond with similarly occurring variations in the factors that underlie the amount of hæmoglobin and the number of corpuscles.

More recent authors, in particular Hammerschlag,

v. Jaksch, v. Limbeck, Biernacki, Dunin, E. Grawitz,
A. Loewy, have avoided an omission of many earlier
investigators; for besides the estimation of the specific
gravity of the total blood, they have carried out that
of one at least of its constituents, either of the corpuscles or of the serum. The red blood corpuscles
have consistently shewn themselves as almost exclusively
concerned with variations in the specific gravity of the
total blood; partly by variations in number, or changes
in their distribution; partly by their chemical instability;
loss of water and absorption of water, and variations in
the amount of iron.

The plasma of the blood on the contrary—and there
is no essential difference between plasma and serum
(Hammerschlag)—is much more constant. Even in severe
pathological conditions, in which the total blood has
become much lighter, the serum preserves its physiological constitution, or undergoes but relatively slight
variations in consistence. Considerable diminutions in
the specific gravity of the serum are much less frequently
observed in primary blood diseases, than in chronic kidney
diseases, and disturbances of the circulation. E. Grawitz
has lately recorded that in certain anæmias, especially
post-hæmorrhagic and those following inanition, the
specific gravity of the serum undergoes perceptible
diminutions[1].

There are still therefore many contradictions in
these results, and it is evidently necessary in a scientific
investigation always to give the specific gravity of the

---

[1] In conditions of shock experimentally produced, the specific gravity
of the total blood is increased, that of the plasma, however, is diminished
(Roy and Cobbett).

serum and of the corpuscles, in addition to that of the total blood.

A method closely related to the estimation of the specific gravity is the direct estimation of the dried substance of the total blood, "HYGRÆMOMETRY"; the clinical introduction of which we owe to Stintzing and Gumprecht. This method is really supplementary to those so far mentioned, and like them can be carried out with the small amounts of blood obtainable at the bedside without difficulty.    Small quantities of blood are received in weighed glass vessels : which are then weighed, dried at 65°—70° C. for 24 hours and then weighed again.    The figures so obtained for the dried substance have a certain independent importance; for they do not run quite parallel with those of the specific gravity, amount of hæmoglobin or number of corpuscles.    The normal values are, for men 21·26 %, for women 19·8 %.

A further procedure for obtaining indirect evidence of the amount of hæmoglobin is the DETERMINATION OF THE VOLUME OF BLOOD CORPUSCLES IN 100 PARTS OF TOTAL BLOOD.    For this estimation a method is desirable, which allows of the separation of the corpuscles from plasma in blood, that is as far as possible unaltered.    The older methods do not fulfil this requirement; since they recommend either defibrination of the blood (quite impossible with the quantities of blood which are generally clinically available); or keeping it fluid by the addition of sodium oxalate or other substances which prevent coagulation. The separation of the two constituents can be effected by simply allowing the blood to settle, or with the centrifugal machine, specially constructed for the blood by Blix-Hedin and Gärtner ("Hæmatocrit").

For these methods various diluting fluids are used,

such as physiological saline solution, $2 \cdot 5 \%$ of potassium bichromate and many others. According to H. Koeppe they are not indifferent as far as the volume of the red blood corpuscles is concerned; and a solution which does not affect the cells must be previously ascertained for each specimen of blood. For this reason attention may be called to the proceeding of M. Herz, in which the clotting of the blood in the pipette is prevented by rendering the walls absolutely smooth by the application of cod-liver oil. Koeppe has slightly varied this method; he fills his handily constructed pipette, very carefully cleaned, with cedar wood oil, and sucks up the blood, as it comes from the fingerprick into the filled pipette. The blood displaces the oil, and as it only comes into contact with perfectly smooth surfaces, it remains fluid. By means of a centrifugal machine, of which he has constructed a very convenient variation, the oil as the lighter body is completely removed from the blood; and the plasma is also separated from the corpuscles. Three sharply defined layers are then visible, the layer of oil above, the plasma layer, and the layer of the red blood corpuscles. In as much as the apparatus is calibrated, the relation between the volumes of the plasma and corpuscles can be read off. No microscopical alterations in the corpuscles are to be observed.

Though this procedure seems very difficult of execution, it is nevertheless the only one, which has really advanced clinical pathology. The results of Koeppe —not as yet very numerous—give the total volume of the red corpuscles as $51 \cdot 1$—$54 \cdot 8 \%$, an average of $52 \cdot 6 \%$.

M. and L. Bleibtreu have endeavoured indirectly to ascertain the relation of the volume of the corpuscles to that of the plasma. Mixtures of blood with physiological saline solution in various proportions are made, in each the amount of nitrogen in the fluid which is left after the corpuscles have settled is estimated. With the aid of quantities so obtained they calculate mathematically the volume of the serum and corpuscles respectively. Apart from the fact that a dilution with salt solution is also here involved, this method is too complicated and requires amounts of blood too large for clinical purposes. Th. Pfeiffer has tried to introduce it clinically in suitable cases, but has not so far succeeded in obtaining definite results. That, however, the relations between the relative volume of the red corpuscles and quantity of hæmoglobin are by no means constant, is well shewn by conditions (for example the acute anæmias) in which an "acute swelling" of the individual red discs occurs (M. Herz), but without a corresponding increase in hæmoglobin. The same conclusion results from recent observations of v. Limbeck, that in catarrhal jaundice a considerable increase of volume of the red blood corpuscles comes to pass under the influence of the salts of the bile acids.

As we have several times insisted, the quantity of hæmoglobin affords the most important measure of the severity of an anæmic condition. Those methods which neither directly nor indirectly give an indication of the amount of hæmoglobin are only so far of interest that they possibly afford an elucidation of the special pathogenesis of blood diseases in particular cases. To these belong the ESTIMATION OF THE ALKALINITY OF THE BLOOD, which in spite of extended observations has not yet obtained importance in the pathology of the blood.

A value to which perhaps attention will be more directed than it has up to the present time by clinicians is the RATE OF COAGULATION OF THE BLOOD, for which comparative results may be obtained by Wright's handy apparatus, the " Coagulometer." In certain conditions, particularly in acute exanthemata, and in the various forms of the hæmorrhagic diathesis, the clotting time is distinctly increased, or indeed clotting may remain in abeyance. Occasionally a distinct acceleration in the clotting, compared with the normal, may be observed. Wright has further ascertained in his excellent researches, that the clotting time can be influenced by drugs : calcium chloride, carbonic acid raise, citric acid, alcohol and increased respiration diminish the clotting power of the blood.

Recently Hayem has repeatedly called attention to a condition, that is probably closely connected with the coagulability of the blood. Although coagulation has set in, the separation of the SERUM FROM THE CLOT occurs only very slightly or not at all. Hayem asserts, that he has found such blood in Purpura hæmorrhagica, Anæmia perniciosa protopathica, malarial cachexia : and some infectious diseases.

For such observations large amounts of blood are needed, which are clinically not frequently available. Certain precautions must be observed, as has been ascertained in the preparation of diphtheria serum, so that the yield of serum may be the largest possible. Amongst these that the blood should be received in longish vessels, which must be especially carefully cleaned, and free from all traces of fat. If the blood-clot does not spontaneously retract it must be freed from the side of the glass with a flat instrument like a paper-knife without injuring it. If no clot occurs in the cold, a result may perhaps follow at blood temperature.

In spite however of all artifices and all care, it is here and there, under pathological conditions, impossible to obtain even a trace of serum from considerable amounts of blood. In a horse for example which was immunised against diphtheria, and had before yielded an unusually large quantity of serum, Ehrlich was able to obtain from 22 kg. of blood scarcely 100 cc. serum, when the animal was bled on account of a tetanus infection.

Perhaps a larger *rôle* is to be allotted in the diseases of the blood to these conditions. Hayem already turns the incomplete production of serum to account, for distinguishing protopathic pernicious anæmia from other severe anæmic conditions. A bad prognosis too may be made when for example in cachetic states this phenomenon is to be observed.

A few methods still remain to be mentioned which test THE RESISTANCE OF THE RED BLOOD CORPUSCLES to external injuries of various kinds.

Landois, Hamburger and v. Limbeck ascertain for instance the degree of concentration of a salt solution, in which the red corpuscles are preserved (" isotonic concentration," Hamburger) and those which cause an exit of the hæmoglobin from the stroma. The erythrocytes are the more resistant, the weaker the concentration which leaves them still uninjured.

Laker tests the red blood corpuscles as regards their resistance to the electric discharge from a Leyden jar, and measures it by the number of discharges up to which the blood in question remains uninjured.

Clinical observation has not yet gained much by these methods. So much only is certain, that in certain diseases: anæmia, hæmoglobinuria, and after many intoxications, the resistance, as measured by the methods above indicated, is considerably lowered.

# THE

# MORPHOLOGY OF THE BLOOD.

# A.  METHODS OF INVESTIGATION.

A GLANCE at the history of the microscopy of the blood shews that it falls into two periods.   In the first, which is especially distinguished by the work of Virchow and Max Schultze, a quantity of positive knowledge was quickly won, and the different forms of anæmia were recognised. But close upon this followed a standstill, which lasted for some decades, the cause of which lay in the circumstance that observers confined themselves to the examination of fresh blood.   What in fact was to be seen with the aid of this simple method, these distinguished observers had quickly exhausted.   That these methods were inadequate is best shewn by the history of leucocytosis, which after the precedent of Virchow was in general referred to an increased production on the part of the lymphatic glands ; and further by the imperfect distinction between leuco- cytosis and incipient leukæmia, which was drawn almost exclusively from purely numerical estimations.   It was only after Ehrlich had introduced the new methods of investigation by means of stained dry preparations, that the histology of the blood received the impulse for its second period.

We owe to them the exact distinction between the several kinds of white blood corpuscles, a rational definition of leukæmia, polynuclear leucocytosis, and the knowledge of the appearances of degeneration and regeneration of the red blood corpuscles, and of their degeneration in hæmo-globinæmic conditions. The same process, then, has gone on in the microscopy of the blood that we see in other branches of normal and pathological histology: by advances in method, advances in knowledge full of importance result. It is therefore little comprehensible, that an author quite recently should recommend a reversion to the old methods, and emphatically announce that he has managed to make a diagnosis in all cases, with the examination of fresh blood. At the present time, after the most important points have been cleared up by new methods, in the large majority of cases, this is not an astonishing achievement. For any difficult case (for instance the early recognition of malignant lymphoma, certain rare forms of anæmia, etc.) as the experienced know, the dry stained preparation is indispensable. The object of examining the blood, is certainly not to make a rapid diagnosis, but to investigate exactly the individual details of the blood picture. To-day, we can only take the standpoint, that everything that is to be seen in fresh specimens—apart from the quite unimportant rouleaux formation, and the amœboid movements—can be seen equally well, and indeed much better in a stained preparation ; and that there are several important details which are only made visible in the latter, and never in wet preparations.

As regards the purely technical side of the question, the examination of stained dry specimens is far more convenient than that of fresh. For it leaves us quite independent of time and place, we can keep the dried blood with few precautions for months at a time, before proceeding to further microscopic treatment; and the examination of the preparation may last as long as required, and can be repeated at any time. On the contrary, the examination of the wet preparation is only possible at the bedside, and must be conducted within so short a time, on account of the changeability of the blood, clotting, destruction of white corpuscles and so forth, that a searching investigation cannot be undertaken. In addition the preparation and staining of dried blood specimens is amongst the simplest and most convenient of the methods of clinical histology. In the interest of its wider dissemination, it will be justifiable to describe it more in detail.

We must also mention here the use of the dry preparation in the estimation of the important relation between the number of the red and of the white corpuscles ; and also of the relative numbers of different kinds of white blood corpuscles.

For this purpose, faultless specimens, specially regularly spread, are indispensable. Quadratic ocular diaphragms (Ehrlich-Zeiss) are requisite, which form a series, so that the sides of the squares are as $1:2:3\ldots\ldots:10$, the fields therefore as $1:4:9\ldots\ldots:100$. The eye-piece made by Leitz after Ehrlich's directions is more convenient, in which, by a handy device, definite square fractions of the field can be obtained. The enumeration is made as follows. The white blood corpuscles are first counted in any desired field with the diaphragm no. 10, that is with the area of 100. Without changing the field, the diaphragm 1, which only leaves free a hundredth part of this area, is now put in, and the red corpuscles are counted. The field is then changed at random, and the red corpuscles counted in a portion of the area which represents the hundredth of that of the white. About 100 such counts are to be made in a specimen. The average of the red corpuscles is then multiplied by 100 and so placed in proportion with the sum of the white. If the white corpuscles are very numerous, so that counting each one in a large field is inconvenient, smaller sections of the eye-piece 81, 64, 49, etc. may be taken.

The important estimation of the percentage relation of the various forms of leucocytes is effected by the simple "typing" of several hundred cells, a count which for the practised observer is completed in less than a quarter of an hour.

## α. **Preparation of the dry specimen.**

To obtain unexceptionable preparations cover-slips of particular quality are necessary. They should not be thicker than 0·08 to 0·10 mm., the glass must not be brittle or faulty, and must in this thickness easily allow of considerable bending, without breaking. Every unevenness of the slip renders it useless for our purposes. The glasses must previously be particularly carefully cleaned, and all fat removed. It is generally sufficient to allow the slips to remain in ether for about half-an-hour, not covering one another. Each one still wet with ether is then wiped with soft, not coarse, linen rag or with tissue-paper. The slips now are put into alcohol for a few minutes, are dried in the same manner as from the ether, and are kept ready for use in a dust-tight watch-glass. Bearing in mind, that these cover-slips are not cut out from a flat piece but from the surface of a sphere, it is evident that only with glasses thus prepared, can it be expected that a capillary space should be formed between two of them, in which the blood spreads easily. For with the smallest unevenness or brittleness of the glass it is an impossibility for the one to fit every bend of the other. And it is only then that the slips can be drawn away one from another, without using a force which breaks them.

To avoid fresh soiling of the cover-slips, and above all the contact of the blood with the moisture coming from the finger, the cover-glass is held with forceps[1] to receive the blood. We recommend for the under cover-glass a clamp forceps $a$, with broad, smooth blades ; the ends may be covered with leather or blotting-paper for a distance of about $\frac{1}{2}$ in. For the other cover-slip a very light spring forceps $b$, with smooth blades, sharp at the tips, is used, with which a cover-glass can be easily picked up from a flat surface. The lower slip is now fixed by one edge in the clamp forceps, and held ready in the left hand. The right hand applies the upper glass with the forceps $b$ to the drop of blood as it exudes from the puncture, and takes it up, without touching the finger itself. The forceps $b$ is then quickly brought to $a$ and the slip with the little drop of blood allowed to fall lightly on the other. In glasses of the right quality the drop distributes itself spontaneously in a completely regular capillary layer. With two fingers of the right hand on the edge of the upper glass, it is now carefully pulled from the lower, which remains fixed in the clamp, without pressing or lifting. Frequently only one, the lower, shews a regular layer, but occasionally both are available for examination. During the desiccation in the air, generally complete in 10—30 seconds, the preparations must naturally be protected from any dampness (for example the breath of the patient).

The extent of surface which is covered depends on the size of the drop, the smaller the latter, the smaller the surface over which it has to be spread. Large drops are quite useless, for with them, the one cover-glass swims on the other, instead of adhering to it.

Although a written description of these manipulations makes the method seem rather intricate, yet but little practice is required to obtain an easy and sure mastery over it. We have felt compelled to describe the method minutely, since preparations so often come under our notice which, although made by scientific men, who pursue hæmatological investigations, are only to be described as technically completely inadequate.

The specimens so obtained, after they are completely dried in the air, should be kept between layers of filter-paper in well closed vessels till further treatment. In important cases, preparations of which it is desirable to keep for some considerable time, some of the specimens should be kept from atmospheric influences by covering

---

[1] Klönne and Müller, Berlin, supply these after Ehrlich's directions.

them with a layer of paraffin. The paraffin must be removed by toluol before proceeding further. The preparations must naturally be kept in the dark.

### β. Fixation of the dry specimen.

All methods of staining available for the blood require the fixing of the proteids of the blood. A general formula cannot be given, since the intensity of the fixation must be regulated in accordance with the kind of stain that is chosen. Relatively slight degrees of hardening suffice for staining in simple watery solutions, for example, in the triacid fluid, and can be attained by a short, and not too intense action of several reagents. For other methods, in which solutions that are strongly acid or alkaline are employed, it is however necessary to fix the structure much more strongly. But here, too, an excess as well as an insufficiency must be guarded against. It is easy with the few staining fluids that are in use to ascertain the optimum for each.

The following means of fixation are employed.

### 1. Dry Heat.

A simple plate of copper on a stand is used, under one end of which burns a Bunsen flame. After some time a certain constancy in the temperature of the plate is reached, the part nearest to the flame is hottest, that farther away is cooler. By dropping water, toluol, xylol, etc. on to it, one can fairly easily ascertain that point of the plate which has reached the boiling temperature of the particular fluid.

Far more convenient is Victor Meyer's apparatus, used by chemists. This consists of a copper boiler, modified for our purpose, with a roof of thin copper-plate, perforated for the opening of the vapour tube. Small quantities of toluol are allowed to boil for a few minutes in the boiler, and the copper-plate soon reaches the temperature of 107°—110°.

For the ordinary staining reagents (in watery fluids) it is enough to place the air-dried preparation at about 110° C. for one half to two minutes. For differential staining mixtures, for instance the eosin-aurantia-nigrosin mixture, a time of two hours is necessary, or higher temperatures must be employed.

## 2. Chemical means.

*a.* To obtain a good triacid stain, the preparations may be hardened, according to Nikiforoff, in a mixture of absolute alcohol and ether of equal parts, for two hours. The beauty of specimens fixed by heat is however not quite fully reached by this method.

*b.* Absolute alcohol fixes dried specimens in five minutes sufficiently to stain them subsequently with Chenzinsky's fluid, or hæmatoxylin-eosin solution. It is an advantage in many cases, especially when rapid investigation is required, to boil the dried preparation in a test-tube in absolute alcohol for one minute.

*c.* Formalin in 1 % alcoholic solution was first used by Benario for fixing blood preparations. The fixation is complete in one minute, and the granulations can be demonstrated. Benario recommends this method of fixing, especially for the hæmatoxylin-eosin staining.

These methods are described as the most suitable

for blood-investigation in general. For special purposes, for instance, the demonstration of mitoses, blood platelets, etc., other hardening reagents may be used with advantage: Sublimate, osmic acid, Flemming's fluid, and so forth.

### γ. Staining of the dry specimen.

Staining methods may be classified according to the purpose to which they are adapted.

We use first those which are suitable for a simple general view. For this it is sufficient to use such solutions as stain hæmoglobin and nuclei simultaneously. (Hæmatoxylin-eosin, hæmatoxylin-orange.)

Occasionally a stain is desirable which only brings out, but in a characteristic manner, a special kind of cell, e.g. the eosinophils, mast cells, or bacteria. Single staining is attained on the principle of maximal decoloration. (Cp. E. Westphal.)

Finally, we have panoptic staining; that is, by methods which bring out, as characteristically as possible, the greatest number of elements. Although we must use high magnifications with these stains, we are compensated by a knowledge of the blood condition that cannot be reached in any other way. A double stain is generally insufficient, and at least three different dyes are used.

Successive staining was formerly used for this purpose. But everyone who has used this method knows how difficult it is to get constant results, however careful one may be in the concentration and time of action of the stain.

Simultaneous staining offers undoubted and important advantages. As there is much obscurity with regard to the

principle on which it rests we may here shortly explain
the theory of simultaneous staining.

We will begin with the simplest example : the use of
picro-carmine, a mixture of neutral ammonium carmine
and ammonium picrate. In a tissue rich in protoplasm,
carmine alone stains diffusely, though the nuclei are
clearly brought out. But if we add an equally concentrated solution of ammonium picrate, the staining gains
extraordinarily in distinctness, in as much as now certain
parts are pure yellow, others pure red. The best known
example is the staining of muscle with picro-carmine, by
which the muscle substance appears pure yellow, the
nuclei pure red. If, however, instead of ammonium
picrate we add another nitro dye which contains more
nitro-groups than picric acid, for example the ammonium
salt of hexa-nitro-diphenylamine, the carmine stain is
completely abolished, all parts stain in the pure aurantia
colour. The explanation of this phenomenon is obvious.
Myosin has a greater affinity for ammonium picrate than
for the carmine salt, and therefore in a mixture of the two
combines with the yellow dye. Owing to this combination it is not now in a condition to chemically fix even
carmine. Further, the nuclei have a great affinity for
the carmine, and therefore stain pure red in this process.
If, however, nitro dyes be added to the carmine solution,
which have an affinity for all tissues, and also for the
nuclei, the sphere of action of the carmine becomes
continually smaller, and finally by the addition of the
most powerful nitro body, the hexa-nitro compound, is
completely abolished. Connective tissue and bone substance, however, behave differently with the picro-carmine
mixture, in as much as here the diffuse stain depends
exclusively on the concentration of the carmine, and is

quite uninfluenced by the addition of a chemical antidote. This staining can only be limited by dilution, but not by the addition of opposed dyes. We must look upon the latter kind of tissue stain not as a chemical combination, but as a mechanical attraction of the stain on the part of the tissue. We may also say: chemical stains are to be recognised by the fact that they react to chemical antidotes; mechanical stains to physical influences; of course always assuming, that purely neutral solutions are employed, and that all additions, which alter the chemical relation of the tissues such as alkalis and acids, or which raise or limit the affinity of the dye for the tissues, are avoided. A further consequence of this view is, that all successive double staining may be serviceably replaced by simultaneous multiple staining, if the chemical nature of the staining process is settled. In contradistinction, in all double stains, which can only be effected by successive staining, mechanical factors are concerned.

In the staining of the dry blood specimen, purely chemical staining processes are concerned, and therefore the polychromatic combination stain is possible in all cases.

The following combinations are possible for the blood:

1. Combined staining with acid dyes. The best known example is the eosin-aurantia-nigrosin mixture, in which the hæmoglobin takes on an orange, the nuclei a black, and the acidophil granulations a red hue.

2. Mixtures of basic dyes. It is possible straight away to make mixtures consisting of two basic dyes. As specially suitable we must mention fuchsin, methyl green, methyl violet, methylene blue. On the other hand, mixtures of three bases are fairly difficult to prepare, and the

quantitative relations of the constituents must be exactly observed. For such mixtures, fuchsin, bismarck brown, chrome green, may be used.

3. Neutral mixtures. These have played an important part in general histology, from the time that they were first introduced by Ehrlich into the histology of the blood up to the present day; and deserve before all others a full consideration.

Neutral staining rests on the fact, that nearly all basic dyes (*i.e.* salts of the dye bases, for instance, rosanilin acetate) form combinations with acid dyes (*i.e.* salts of the dye acids, for instance, ammonium picrate) which are to be regarded as neutral dyes, such as rosanilin picrate. Their employment offers considerable difficulties as they are very imperfectly soluble in water. A practical application of them was first possible after Ehrlich had ascertained that certain series of the neutral dyes are easily soluble in excess of the acid dye, and so the preparation of solutions of the required strength, readily kept, was made possible. Among the basic dyes which are suitable for this purpose are those particularly which contain the ammonium group, especially methyl green, methylene blue, amethyst violet[1] (tetraethylsafraninchloride), and to a certain extent pyronin and rhodamin also. In contradistinction to these, the members of the triphenylmethan series, such as fuchsin, methyl violet, bismarck brown, phosphin, indazine, are in general less suited for the purpose, with the exception of methyl green already mentioned. The acid dyes specially suited for the production of soluble neutral stains are the easily soluble salts of the polysulpho-acids. The salts of the carbonyl acids and other acid phenol dyes are but little

---

[1] Baden Anilin and Soda manufactory, Kalle and Co.

suitable: and least of all, the nitro dyes. Specially to be mentioned among the acid dye series are those which can be used for the preparation of the neutral mixtures: orange g., acid fuchsin, narcëin (an easy soluble yellow dye, the sodium salt of sulphanilic acid—hydrazo—β-naphtholsulphonic acid).

If a solution of methyl green be allowed to fall drop by drop into a solution of an acid dye, for instance orange g., a coarse precipitate first results, which dissolves completely on the further addition of the orange. No more orange should be added than is necessary for complete solution. This is the type of a simple neutral staining fluid. Chemically the above-mentioned example may be thus explained; in this mixture all three basic groups of the methyl green are united with the acid dye, so that we have produced a triacid compound of methyl green.

Simple neutral mixtures, which have one constituent in common, may be combined together straight away. This is very important for triple staining, which can only be attained by mixing together two simple neutral mixtures, each consisting of two components. A chemical decomposition need not be feared. We thus get mixtures containing three and more colours. Theoretically there are two possibilities for such combinations:

1. Staining mixtures of 1 acid and 2 basic dyes,

*e.g.*  orange — amethyst — methyl green;
narcëin — pyronin — methyl green;
narcëin — pyronin — methylene blue.

2. Staining mixtures of 2 acids and 1 base, in particular the mixture to be described later in detail of

orange g. — acid fuchsin — methyl green.
Further narcëin — acid fuchsin — methyl green,

and the corresponding combinations with methylene blue, and amethyst violet may be mentioned.

The importance of these neutral staining solutions lies in the fact that they pick out definite substances, which would not be demonstrated by the individual components, and which we therefore call neutrophil.

Elements which have an affinity for basic dyes, such as nuclear substances, stain in these neutral mixtures purely in the colour of the basic dye; acidophil elements in that of one of the two acid dyes; whilst those portions of tissue which from their constitution have an equal affinity for acid and basic dyes, attract the neutral compound, as such, and therefore stain in the mixed colour.

The eosine-methylene blue mixtures are exceptional in so far, that it is possible with them, for a short time at least, to preserve active solutions, in which with an excess of basic methylene blue, enough eosin is dissolved for both to come into play. A drawback however of such mixtures is, that in them precipitates are very easily produced, which render the preparation quite useless. This danger is particularly great in freshly prepared solutions. In solutions, such as Chenzinsky's, which can be kept active for a longer time, it is less. Hence fresh solutions stain far more intensely and more variously than older ones, and are therefore used in special cases (see page 46). If the stain is successful the appearances are very instructive. Nuclei are blue, hæmoglobin red, neutrophil granulation violet, acidophil pure red, mast cell granulation deep blue, forming one of the most beautiful microscopic pictures.

For practical purposes, besides the iodine and iodine-eosine solution described below (see page 46) the following are especially used:

1. Hæmatoxylin solution with eosin or orange g.

| | |
|---|---|
| Eosin (cryst.) | 0·5 |
| Hæmatoxylin | 2·0 |
| Alcohol abs. | |
| Aqu. dest. | |
| Glycerine *aa* | 100·0 |
| Glacial acetic acid | 10·0 |
| Alum in excess | |

The fluid must stand for some weeks. The preparations, fixed in absolute alcohol, or by short heating, stain in from half-an-hour to two hours. The hæmoglobin and eosinophil granules are red, the nuclei stain in the colour of hæmatoxylin. The solution must be very carefully washed off.

2. In the practical application of the triacid fluid, particular care must be taken, as M. Heidenhain first shewed, that the dyes are chemically pure[1]. Formerly granules, apparently basophil, were frequently observed in the white blood corpuscles, particularly in the region of the nucleus. They were not recognised, even by practised observers (*e.g.* Neusser) as artificial, but were regarded as preformed, and were described as perinuclear forms. Since the employment of pure dyes these appearances, whose meaning for a long time puzzled us, are but seldom seen.

Saturated watery solutions of the three dyes are first prepared, and cleared by standing for some considerable time. The following mixture is now made:

| | |
|---|---|
| 13—14 c.c. | Orange-g. solution |
| 6—7 c.c. | Acid fuchsin solution |

[1] At M. Heidenhain's instigation, the Anilin-dye Company of Berlin have prepared the three dyes in the crystalline form.

| 15 c.c. | Aqu. dest. |
| 15 c.c. | Alcohol |
| 12·5 c.c. | Methyl green |
| 10 c.c. | Alcohol |
| 10 c.c. | Glycerine |

These fluids are measured in the above-mentioned order, with the same measuring glass; and from the addition of methyl green onwards the fluid is thoroughly shaken. The solution can be used at once, and keeps indefinitely. The staining of the blood specimen in triacid requires only a little fixation, cp. page 35. The stain is completed in five minutes at most.

The nuclei are greenish, the red blood corpuscles orange, the acidophil granulation copper red, the neutrophil violet. The mast cells stand out by " negative staining " as peculiar bright, almost white cells, with nuclei of a pale green colour.

The triacid stain is very convenient. It is much to be recommended for good general preparations; it is indispensable in all cases where the study of the neutrophil granulations is concerned.

3. Basic double staining. Saturated, watery methyl-green solution is mixed with alcoholic fuchsin.

The stain, which only requires a small fixation, is completed in a few minutes, and colours the nuclei green, the red blood corpuscles red, the protoplasm of the leucocytes fuchsin colour. It is therefore specially suited for demonstration preparations of lymphatic leukæmia.

4. Eosin-methylene blue mixtures, for example Chenzinsky's fluid:

| Concentrated watery methylene blue solution | 40 c.c. |
| $\frac{1}{2}$ % eosin solution in 70 % alcohol | 20 c.c. |
| Aqua dest. | 40 c.c. |

This fluid is fairly stable, but must always be filtered before use. It only requires a fixation of the specimen for five minutes in absolute alcohol. The staining takes 6–24 hours (in air-tight watch-glasses) at blood temperature. The nuclei and the mast cell granulations stain deep blue, malaria plasmodia light sky blue, red corpuscles and eosinophil granules a fine red.

This solution is particularly suited for the study of the nuclei, the baso and eosinophil granulations, and it is used by preference for anæmic blood, and also for lymphatic leukæmia.

5. 10 c.c. of a 1 per cent. watery eosin solution, with 8 c.c. methylal, and 10 c.c. of a saturated watery solution of methylene blue are mixed, and used at once, see page 41. Time of staining 1, at most 2 minutes. The staining is characteristic only in preparations very carefully fixed by heat. The mast cell granulations are stained pure blue, the eosinophil red, the neutrophil in mixed colour.

6. Jenner's stain consists of a solution in methyl alcohol of the precipitate formed by adding eosine to methylene blue.

Grubler's water soluble eosine, yellow $1\cdot25\%$ ⎫ a.a. watery
      „    medicinal, methylene blue $1\%$ ⎭ solutions.

Precipitate allowed to stand 24 hours, and then dried at 55°. It is then made up to $\frac{1}{2}\%$ in methyl alcohol (Merck). The stain may be obtained from R. Kanthack, 18, Berners Street, London, ready for use. It is exceedingly sensitive to acids and alkalis. Fixation is effected by heat. Time of staining 1–4 minutes.

Before we pass to the histology of the blood, two important methods may be described, for which the dried blood preparation is employed directly, without previous fixation: 1. the recognition of glycogen in the blood; 2. the microscopic test of the distribution of the alkali of the blood.

### 1. *Recognition of glycogen in blood.*

This may be effected in two ways. The original procedure consisted in putting the preparation into a drop of thick cleared iodine-indiarubber solution under the microscope, as had been already recommended by Ehrlich for the recognition of glycogen.

The following method is still better. The preparation is placed in a closed vessel containing iodine crystals. Within a few minutes it takes on a dark brown colour, and is then mounted in a saturated lævulose solution, whose index of refraction is very high. To preserve these specimens they must be surrounded with some kind of cover-glass cement.

By the use of better methods the red blood corpuscles which have taken on the iodine stain stand out, without having undergone any morphological change. The white blood corpuscles are only slightly stained. All parts containing glycogen on the contrary, whether the glycogen be in the white blood corpuscles, or extracellular, are characterised by a beautiful mahogany brown colour. The second modification of this method is specially to be recommended on account of the strong clearing action of the lævulose syrup. In using the iodine-indiarubber solution a small quantity of glycogen in the cells may escape observation owing to the opaqueness of the india-rubber, and occasionally too by the separate staining of the same. The second more delicate method is for this reason recommended, in the investigation of cases of diabetes and other diseases [1].

2. The microscopic test of the distribution of alkali in the blood.

These methods rest on a procedure of Mylius for the estimation of the amount of alkali in glass. Iodine-eosine is a red compound easily soluble in water, which is not soluble in ether, chloroform, or toluol. But the free coloured acid, which is precipitated by acidifying solutions of the salt, is very sparingly soluble in water. It is, on the contrary, very easily soluble in organic solvents, so that by shaking, it completely passes over into an etherial solution, which becomes yellow. If this solution be allowed to fall on glass, on which deposits of alkali have been formed by decomposition, they stand out in a fine red colour as the result of the production of the deeply coloured salt.

In its application to the blood, of course the vessels used for staining as well as the cover-glasses must be cleaned from all adhering traces of alkali by means of acids. The dry specimen is thrown directly after its preparation into a glass vessel containing a chloroform or chloroform-toluol solution of free iodine-eosine. In a short time it becomes dark red. It is then quickly transferred to another vessel containing pure chloroform, which is once more changed, and the preparation still wet from the chloroform is then mounted in canada balsam. In such preparations the morphological elements have preserved

[1] It may also be used for the recognition of glycogen in secretions. For instance, gonorrhœal pus always shews a considerable glycogen reaction of the pus cells. It is found, moreover, in cells which originate from tumours, whether these be present in exudations, or obtained by scraping.

their shape completely. The plasma shews a distinct red colour, whilst the red corpuscles have taken up no colour. The protoplasm of the white corpuscles is red, the nuclei appear as spaces, because unstained (negative nuclear staining). The disintegrated corpuscles and the fibrin which is produced, shew an intense red stain. These stains are peculiarly instructive, and shew many details which are not visible in other methods. The study of these preparations is really of the highest value, since they allow the products of manipulation of the dry preparation and every error of production to stand out in the most reliable manner, and so render possible a kind of automatic control. The scientific value of this method lies in the fact that it throws light on the distribution of the alkali in the individual elements of the blood. It appears that free alkali reacting on iodine-eosine is not present in the nuclei; these must therefore have a neutral or an acid reaction. On the contrary the protoplasm of the leucocytes is always alkaline, and the largest amount of alkali is held by the protoplasm of the lymphocytes. We call particular attention, in this connection, to the strong alkalinity of the blood platelets.

# B. NORMAL AND PATHOLOGICAL HISTOLOGY OF THE BLOOD.

In satisfactorily prepared dry specimens the red blood corpuscles keep their natural size and shape, and their biconcavity is plainly seen. They present a distinct round homogeneous form, of about $7·5\,\mu$ in diameter. They are most intensely coloured in a broad peripheral layer, and most faintly in the centre corresponding to their depression. With all stains mentioned above the stroma is quite uncoloured, and the hæmoglobin exclusively attracts the stain, so that for a practised observer the depth of stain gives a certain indication of the hæmoglobin equivalent of each cell, and a better one than the natural colour of the hæmoglobin in the fresh specimen. Corpuscles poor in hæmoglobin are easily recognised by their fainter staining, especially by the still greater brightness of the central zone. When somewhat more marked, they present appearances which from the isolated staining of the periphery Litten has happily named " pessary " forms. The faint staining of a red corpuscle cannot be explained, as E. Grawitz assumes, by a diminished affinity of the hæmoglobin for the dye. Qualitative changes of this kind of the hæmoglobin, expressing themselves in an altered relationship towards dyes, do not occur, even in anæmic blood. If in the latter, the blood discs stain less intensely, this is due exclusively to the smaller amount of hæmoglobin.

A diminution in the hæmoglobin content can in this way be shewn in all anæmic conditions, especially in posthæmorrhagic, secondary and chlorotic cases. On the contrary, as Laache first observed, in the pernicious anæmias, the hæmoglobin equivalent of the individual discs is raised.

To appreciate correctly pathological conditions, it must always be borne in mind, that in normal blood the individual red blood corpuscles are by no means of the same value. Step by step some of the cells are used up and replaced by new. Every drop of blood contains, side by side, the most various stages of life of fully formed erythrocytes. For this reason influences which affect the blood—provided their intensity does not exceed a certain degree—cannot equally influence all red corpuscles. The least resistant elements, that is, the oldest, will succumb to the effect of influences, to which other and more vigorous cells adapt themselves.

To influences, of this moderate degree, belongs without doubt the anæmic constitution of the blood as such, the effect of which in this direction one can best investigate in cases of posthæmorrhagic anæmia.

In all anæmic conditions we observe characteristic changes in the blood discs.

A. Anæmic or polychromatophil degeneration.
This change in the red blood corpuscles, first described by Ehrlich, to which the second name was given later by Gabritschewski, is only recognisable in stained preparations. The red blood discs, which under normal circumstances stain in pure hæmoglobin colour, now

take on a mixed colour. For instance, the red corpuscles are pure red in preparations of normal blood, stained with hæmatoxylin-eosine mixture. But in preparations of blood of a chromic anæmia stained with the same solution, in which possibly all stages of the degeneration in question are present, one sees red discs with a faint inclination to violet; others which are bluish red; and at the end of the series, forms stained a fairly intense blue, in which scarcely a trace of red can be seen, and which by their peculiar notched periphery are evidently to be regarded as dying elements.

Ehrlich put forward the theory, that this remarkable behaviour towards dyes indicates a gradual death of the red blood corpuscles, that is of the old forms, leading to a coagulation necrosis of the discoplasm. The latter takes up, as is the case in coagulation necrosis, the proteids of the blood, and acquires thereby the power of combining with nuclear stains. At the same time the discoplasm loses its power of retaining the hæmoglobin, and gives it up to the blood plasma in ever increasing quantity as the change proceeds. Hence the disc continues to lose the capacity for the specific hæmoglobin stain.

Objection has been raised to these views from many quarters, especially from Gabritschewski, and afterwards from Askanazy, Dunin and others. The polychromatophil discs are not, they say, dying forms, but on the contrary represent young individuals. The circumstance, that in certain anæmias the early stages of the nucleated red corpuscles are variously polychromatic, was evidence for this opinion.

In view of the great theoretical importance which

attaches to this subject, the grounds for regarding this change as degenerative, may be here shortly brought forward.

1. The appearance of the erythrocytes which shew polychromatophilia in the highest degree. By the notching of their margins they appear to eyes practised in the judgment of morphological conditions, in a stage almost of dissolution, and as well-pronounced degeneration forms.

2. The fact that by animal experiment, for instance, in inanition, their appearance in large numbers in the blood can be produced. That is, precisely in conditions, where there can be least question of a fresh production of red blood corpuscles.

3. The clinical experience, that in acute losses of blood in man, these staining anomalies, can be observed in numerous cells, within so short a time as the first 24 hours. Whilst in our observations, which are very numerous upon this point, embracing several hundred cases, and carried out with particular care, no nucleated red blood corpuscles in this space of time can be found in man[1].

4. The polychromatophil degeneration can frequently be observed in nucleated red blood corpuscles, particularly in the megaloblasts. This fact can be so easily established that it can hardly escape even an unpractised observer, and it was sufficiently familiar to Ehrlich, who first directed attention to these conditions. The fact that the normoblasts, which are typical of normal regeneration,

---

[1] Dunin, on the contrary, designates the appearance of nucleated red blood corpuscles within the first 24 hours after the loss of blood as normal and regular. This view does not correspond with the facts. A single case on one occasion may exhibit a rarity of this kind.

are as a rule free from polychromatophil degeneration, gave the key for the interpretation of this appearance. And similarly for the nucleated red blood corpuscles of lower animals. Askanazy asserts that the nucleated red blood corpuscles of the bone-marrow, which he was able to investigate in a case of empyema, shew, immediately after the resection of the ribs, complete polychromatophilia. This perhaps depends on the peculiarities of the case, or on the uncertainty of the staining method: eosine-methylene blue stain, which is for this purpose very unreliable, since slight overstaining towards blue readily occurs. (We expressly advise the use of the triacid solution or of the hæmatoxylin-eosine mixture for the study of the anæmic degenerations.)

After what has been adduced, we hold in agreement with the recent work of Pappenheim, and Maragliano, that the appearance of polychromatophilia is a sign of degeneration. To explain the presence of erythroblasts which have undergone these changes we must suppose that in severe injuries to the life of the blood these elements are not produced in the usual fashion, but from the very beginning are morbidly altered. Analogies from general pathology suggest themselves in sufficient number.

B. A second change that we find in the red blood corpuscles of the anæmias, is poikilocytosis.

By this name a change of the blood is denoted, where along with normal red blood corpuscles, larger, smaller and minute red elements are found in greater or less number. The excessively large cells are found in pernicious anæmia, as Laache first observed, and as has since been generally confirmed. On the contrary in all other severe or moderate anæmic conditions, the red corpuscles shew a diminution in volume, and in their amount of hæmoglobin. This contradiction, which Laache first mentioned, but was unable to explain, has found a satisfactory solution in Ehrlich's researches on the nucleated precursors of the myelocytes and normocytes (see below).

The blood picture of the anæmias is made still more complicated in that the diminutive cells do not preserve their normal shape, but assume the well-known irregular forms: pear-, balloon-, saucer-, canoe-shapes. Nevertheless in good dry preparations the smallest forms usually still shew the central depression. The so-called "microcytes" constitute an exception to this statement. These are small round forms, to which was allotted in the early days of the microscopic investigation of the blood, a special significance for the severe anæmias. They are however nothing but contraction forms of the poikilocytes, as the crenated are of the normal corpuscles. Consequently microcytes are but seldom found in dried specimens, whilst in wet preparations they are easily seen after some time. It is further of importance to know, that in fresh blood the poikilocytes exhibit certain movements, which have already given rise to mistakes in many ways. Thus at one time the poikilocytes were considered to be the cause of malaria. More recently the somewhat larger sizes were regarded by Klebs, Perles as amœbæ and similar organisms. In agreement with Hayem, who from the very first described these forms as pseudo-parasites, a warning must be given against attributing a parasitic character to them.

The origin of poikilocytosis, previously the subject of

much discussion, is now generally explained in Ehrlich's way. For the mere fact, that by careful heating, poikilocytosis can be experimentally produced in any blood, forces one to the assumption that the poikilocytes are products of a fragmentation of the red blood corpuscles ("schistocytes," Ehrlich). And correspondingly the smallest fragments shew the biconcave form in the dry specimen; for they too contain the specific protoplasm of the disc "which possesses the inherent tendency to assume the typical biconcave form in a state of equilibrium."

Qualitative changes in the protoplasm of the poikilocytes are not to be observed, even by staining; and one may therefore ascribe to them complete functional power, and regard their production as a purposeful reaction to the diminished number of corpuscles. For by the division of a larger blood corpuscle into a series of homologous smaller ones, the respiratory surface is considerably increased.

C. A third morphological variation which anæmic blood may shew in the more severe degrees of the disease, is the appearance of nucleated red blood corpuscles.

Though we do not wish to enter here upon the latest questions concerning the origin of the blood elements, we must shortly indicate the present state of our knowledge of the nucleated red corpuscles.

Since the fundamental work of Neumann and Bizzozero, the nucleated forms have been generally recognised as the young stages of the normal red blood corpuscles. Hayem's theory, on the contrary, obstinately asserts the origin of the erythrocytes from blood-platelets, and has, excepting by the originator and his pupils, been generally allowed to drop.

Ehrlich had in the year 1880 pointed out the clinical importance of the nucleated red blood corpuscles, in as much as he demonstrated that in the so-called secondary anæmias, and in leukæmia, nucleated corpuscles of the normal size, " normoblasts "; in pernicious anæmia excessively large elements, "megaloblasts," " gigantoblasts " are present. At the same time Ehrlich mentioned that the megaloblasts also play a prominent part in embryonic blood formation.

In 1883 Hayem likewise proposed a similar division of the nucleated red blood corpuscles into two,

(1) the "globules nuclées géantes" which he found exclusively in the embryonic state, (2) the "globules nuclées de taille moyennes" which he found invariably present in the later stages of embryonic life, and in adults. Further, W. H. Howell (1890) found in cats' embryoes two kinds of erythrocytes, (1) very large, equivalent to the blood cells of reptiles and amphibia ("ancestor corpuscles"), and (2) of the usual size of the blood corpuscles of mammalia. And similarly more recent authors, H. F. Müller, C. S. Engel, Pappenheim and others, have adhered to the division of hæmatoblasts into normo- and megaloblasts. And it is on the whole recognised, that, physiologically, normoblasts are always present in the bone-marrow of adults, as the precursors of the non-nucleated erythrocytes; that the megaloblasts, however, are never found there under normal circumstances, but only in embryonic stages, and in the first years of extra-uterine life.

S. Askanazy on the contrary has expressed the view, that the normoblasts may arise from the megaloblasts, and thereby denies the principal distinction between them. Schaumann also holds that the separation of the two kinds rests on doubtful foundation, since occasionally it is questionable whether particular cells are the normoblasts or the megaloblasts.

We distinguish three kinds of nucleated red blood-corpuscles on the grounds of the following characters;

1. The normoblasts. These are red corpuscles of the size of the usual non-nucleated disc, whose protoplasm as a rule shews a pure hæmoglobin colour, and which possess a nucleus. Occasionally there may be 2—4 nuclei. The sharply defined nucleus lies generally in the centre, comprises the greater part of the cell, and is above all distinguished by its intense colour with nuclear stains, which exceeds that of the nuclei of the leucocytes, and indeed of all known nuclei. This property is so characteristic that the free nuclei, which occur occasionally in anæmias, and particularly often in leukæmia, may be recognised as nuclei of normoblasts, although surrounded by traces only of hæmoglobin, or by none at all.

2. The megaloblasts. These are 2—4 times as large as normal red blood corpuscles. Their protoplasm, which constitutes by far the chief portion of the body of the cell, very often shews anæmic degeneration to a greater or less degree. The nucleus is larger than that of the normoblasts, but does not form so considerable a fraction of the cell as in the latter. It is often not sharply defined, and is of a rounded shape. It is distinguished from the nucleus of the normoblast by its much weaker affinity for nuclear stains, which may often be so small that little practised observers perceive no nucleus.

Occasionally very large cells are present of the kind just described, which are therefore called gigantoblasts, but which are not distinguishable in other respects from the megaloblasts.

It cannot be denied that it is often difficult to decide whether a particular cell is to be regarded as a specially small megaloblast or a large normoblast. In such cases one would naturally search the preparation for perfect forms of hæmatoblasts, and for the presence of free nuclei or of megalocytes, in order to obtain an indirect conclusion concerning the cells in question.

3. The microblasts. These are occasionally present, *e.g.* in traumatic anæmias, but they are very seldom found, and have not so far attracted particular attention.

---

The question of the meaning of the normoblasts and megaloblasts has led to lively and significant discussions, partly in favour of, partly against the distinction between these two cell forms. After surveying the literature, we are forced to separate the megaloblasts from the normoblasts, in the first place because of their subsequent histories, and the peculiarities of their nuclei, and secondly because of clinical observation.

α. The fate of the nuclei. For some time past two views, almost diametrically opposed, have been in existence with regard to the nature of the change of the nucleated to the non-nucleated erythrocytes. The chief exponent of the one, Rindfleisch, taught that the nucleus of the erythroblasts leaves the cell, which thereby becomes a complete erythrocyte, whilst the nucleus itself, by the aid of the small remnant of protoplasm which surrounds it, takes up new material from the surrounding plasma, manufactures hæmoglobin and so becomes a fresh erythroblast.

According to the second theory the erythroblasts change to non-nucleated discs by the destruction and solution of the nucleus within the cell body. ("Karyorrhexis," "Karyolysis.") The authors who support this view and also describe it as the only kind of erythrocyte formation are chiefly Kölliker and E. Neumann.

Rindfleisch arrived at his theory by direct observation of the process described, as it occurred in physiological saline solution with the blood of fœtal guinea-pigs and teased preparations of bone-marrow.

E. Neumann regards Rindfleisch's doctrine as untenable, since the process which he observed is chiefly the result of a severe injury of the blood from the sodium chloride solution and the teasing. If a method of preparation be chosen which protects the blood as far as possible, and avoids every chemical and physical alteration, the exit of the nucleus as described by Rindfleisch does not occur.

The view of Kölliker and Neumann that the nuclei gradually decay in the interior of the cell is not supported by the observation of a process, but by the fact that in suitable material, for instance, fœtal bone-marrow, liver blood, and leukæmic blood, the transition from erythroblast to erythrocyte is shewn by all phases of nuclear metamorphosis. v. Recklinghausen professes to have directly observed the dissolution of the nucleus within the cell in rabbit's blood, kept living in a moist chamber. Pappenheim's opinion however, that in this case processes are concerned such as Maragliano and Castellino have described as artificial necrobiosis, seems in this connection worthy of consideration.

Just as with regard to the formation of erythrocytes the views differ one from another, so also with regard to the "free" nuclei which come under observation in numerous preparations. Kölliker has taught that these nuclei are not quite free, but are always surrounded by a minute border of protoplasm. On the other hand Rindfleisch regards these nuclei as having migrated from, or having been cast off by the erythroblasts; and Neumann explains them as the early forms of erythroblasts. Ehrlich was the first to endeavour to effect a compromise between the directly opposed views of Rindfleisch and Neumann. He taught that both kinds take part in the production of the red discs. From blood preparations which contain numerous normoblasts, for instance in "blood crises" (see p. 62), an unbroken series of pictures can easily be put together shewing how the nucleus of the erythroblast leaves the cell, and at last produces the appearance of the so-called free nucleus. It must be expressly mentioned that these pictures are only to be found in specimens in whose preparation pressure of any kind upon the blood has been avoided. Further, however rich a blood may be in normoblasts, the metamorphosis of the nucleus as described by Neumann, is practically never to be observed. It is quite otherwise with the megaloblasts. Amongst them, few examples are to be found in which traces at least of the destruction and solution of the nucleus are not shewn, and in a blood preparation of pernicious anæmia, which is not too poor in megaloblasts, one can construct step by step the unbroken series from megaloblasts with a complete nucleus through all stages of Karyorrhexis and Karyolysis to the megalocytes, as the process is described by Neumann[1].

[1] Probably the dot-like and granular enclosures in the red corpuscles, which stain with methylene blue, and which Askanzy and A. Lazarus

From Ehrlich's observations it follows, that the normo-blasts become normocytes by extrusion or emigration of the nucleus, the megaloblasts become megalocytes by degeneration of the nucleus within the cell.

M. B. Schmidt without making use of the principal distinction made by Ehrlich, also concludes from his researches on sections of the bone-marrow of animals in extra-uterine life, that both kinds of erythrocyte formation occur.

Quite recently Pappenheim, partly in conjunction with O. Israel, has carried out very thorough researches on these particular points. As the subject for observation he chose the blood of embryonic mice. He was able in the first place, like Rindfleisch, to produce the exit of the nuclei from the cells by the addition of "physiological" salt solution to fresh blood, and is of the opinion that the exit of the nucleus from the erythroblasts only takes place artificially.

In embryonic blood the metamorphosis to erythrocytes occurs exclusively by nuclear destruction and solution within the cell, be it in the case of megalo- or giganto-blasts or of cells of the size of the normal red blood corpuscle.

The free nuclei that are observed, whose appearance Pappenheim explains by a preceding solution of the protoplasm (plasmolysis), he regards, in opposition to Rindfleisch and Neumann, not as the beginnings of a developmental series, but as the surviving remnants of the degenerated dying blood cells. Clinical observation, certainly, does not support this conception of Pappen-heim's; in as much as in suitable cases with numerous

have observed in numerous cases of pernicious anæmia are also products of a similar nuclear destruction.

free nuclei (leukæmia, blood crises) transitional forms, which according to Pappenheim must necessarily be present, are not to be found. Moreover, in alluding to a case of leukæmia of this kind, this author himself admits that the appearance of free nuclei can be explained in this instance by the exit of the nucleus.

Although Pappenheim, as above mentioned, recognises no difference between megaloblasts and normoblasts in embryonic blood as far as the fate of the nucleus is concerned, he nevertheless decidedly supports Ehrlich's separation of the erythroblasts into these two groups, as two hæmatogenetically distinct species of cells. He does not regard as distinguishing characteristics, the size and hæmoglobin content of the cells—although as we have described above, these are in general different in normo- and megaloblasts—for these two properties undergo such great variations as to increase considerably under certain circumstances the difficulty of diagnosis of individual cells. The chief characteristic is, as Ehrlich has always particularly insisted, the constitution of the nucleus. The nuclei of cells which are with certainty to be reckoned among the normoblasts are marked by the absence of structure, their sharply defined contour, their intense affinity for nuclear stains. That is by properties which histology sums up under the name Pyknosis (Pfitzner) and recognises as signs of old age. The nuclei of the megaloblasts are round, shew a good deal of structure, and stain far less deeply.

β. The clinical differences. Normoblasts are found almost invariably in all severe anæmias that are the result of trauma, inanition or organic disease of some kind. They are however mostly rather scanty, so that a preparation must be searched for some time before an example is found. But occasionally, most often in acute, but also in chronic anæmias, and even in cachectic conditions, every field shews one or more normoblasts.

V. Noorden was the first to describe a case in which in the course of a hæmorrhagic anæmia normoblasts temporarily appeared in such overwhelming numbers in the circulating blood, that the microscopic picture, which at the same time comprised a marked hyperleucocytosis, was almost similar to that of a myelogenous leukæmia. And as in addition to this occurrence the number of blood corpuscles was nearly doubled, v. Noorden gave it the distinctive name "blood crisis."

The following procedure is to be recommended for the investigation of the blood crisis:

1. Estimation of the absolute number of red blood corpuscles.

2. Estimation of the proportion of white to red corpuscles.

3. Estimation of the proportion of nucleated red to white corpuscles by means of the quadratic ocular diaphragm (see page 31) in the dry preparation.

For instance if we find in a case of anæmia, $3\frac{1}{2}$ millions of red blood corpuscles, the proportion of white to red corpuscles $= \frac{1}{100}$ and that of the nucleated red to the white $= \frac{1}{10}$, then in 1 cubic millimeter there are 3500 nucleated red corpuscles, that is for 1000 ordinary there is 1 nucleated corpuscle.

Megaloblasts on the contrary are never found in traumatic anæmias. And in chronic anæmias of the severest degree, the result for example of old syphilis, carcinoma of the stomach and so forth, one looks for them almost always in vain, although they are sometimes to be found in leukæmia. On the contrary, the conditions, apparently much milder, in which from the clinical history, ætiology and general objective symptoms pernicious anæmia is suggested, are almost without exception characterised by the appearance of megaloblasts in the blood. Nevertheless in very late stages of the disease they are always scanty, and a very tedious search through one or more specimens is often required to demonstrate their presence. Hence follows the rule, that the investigation of a case of severe anæmia should never be considered closed, before three or four preparations at least have been minutely searched for megaloblasts under an oil immersion objective.

This clinical difference between the two kinds of hæmatoblasts admits of but one natural conclusion, which primarily leaves untouched the question, so much discussed at the present time, whether the megalo- or normoblasts can change one to the other. In all cases of anæmia, in which the fresh formation occurs according to the normal type, only in greater quantity and more energetically, we find normoblasts. Almost all anæmias resulting from known causes: acute hæmorrhages, chronic hæmorrhages, poverty of blood from inanition, cachexias, blood poisons, hæmaglobinæmia and so forth,—in short all conditions rightly called, secondary, symptomatic anæmias,—may shew this increase of normal blood production. In the conditions, which Biermer, on the grounds of their clinical peculiarities, has distinguished as "essential, pernicious anæmia" megaloblasts on the contrary occur, and represent an embryonic type of development. The extent to which this type participates in the blood formation in pernicious anæmia is most simply demonstrated by the fact that megaloblasts are present in all cases of pernicious anæmia, as Laache first shewed, and in some cases form the preponderating portion of the blood discs. Whilst, therefore, in the ordinary kinds of anæmia we find that the red corpuscles tend to produce small forms, in pernicious anæmia, on the other hand, and exclusively in this form, we find a tendency in the opposite direction. This constant difference cannot be a chance result, but must depend on some constant law: in pernicious anæmia excessively large blood corpuscles are produced. Ehrlich's demonstration of megaloblasts has sufficed for this logical advance. All researches, which try to obscure or totally deny the distinction between megaloblasts and normoblasts are wrecked by the simple clinical fact that in pernicious anæmia the blood is megaloblastic.

The appearance of megaloblasts and megalocytes is therefore evidence that the regeneration of the blood in the bone-marrow is not proceeding in the normal manner, but in a way which approximates to the embryonic type. The extreme cases are naturally seldom, such as that of Rindfleisch, in which the whole bone-marrow was found full of megaloblasts. It is sufficiently conclusive for the pernicious nature of the case, "if only considerable portions but not the whole marrow, have lapsed into megaloblastic degeneration." We can now say that the megaloblastic metamorphosis is not a purposeful process, and for the following reasons: 1. Since the fresh formation of red blood corpuscles by means of the megaloblastic method is clearly much slower. This is especially borne out by the fact that the megaloblasts are present in the blood always in small numbers only, whilst the normoblasts, as above mentioned, are often found in much larger quantities. In agreement with this, "blood crises" are not to be observed in the megaloblastic anæmias. 2. Since the megalocytes which are formed from the megaloblasts possess in proportion to their volume a relatively smaller respiratory surface, and so constitute a type disadvantageous for anæmic conditions[1]. This is still more evident when we remember that the production of poikilocytes is on the contrary a serviceable process.

The megaloblastic degeneration of the bone-marrow is no doubt due to chemical influences, which alter the type of regeneration in a disadvantageous manner. We do not for the most part yet know the exciting causes of the toxic process; consequently we are unable to put a stop to it, and its termination is lethal. The Bothriocephalus anæmias, which in general as is well-known offer a good prognosis, by no means contradict this view. They hold their privileged position amongst the anæmias of the megaloblastic type, only for the reason that their cause is known to us, and can be removed. As in many infectious diseases, individuals react quite differently to the presence of the Bothriocephalus. Some remain well; others show the signs of simple anæmia, ultimately with normoblasts; whilst a third group presents the typical picture of pernicious anæmia. For many years, so long as its ætiology was unknown, Bothriocephalus anæmia was not separated on clinical grounds from pernicious anæmia. Severe Bothriocephalus anæmia may be described as a pernicious anæmia, with a known and removable cause. Good evidence for this point of view is afforded by a case of Askanazy, who describes a severe pernicious anæmia, with typical megaloblasts, in which after the

---

[1] It does not seem superfluous in this place expressly to emphasise, that what has been said on the diagnostic importance of the megaloblasts only holds for the blood of adults. For the conditions of the blood in children, which vary in many respects from that of adults see "Die Anæmie," Ehrlich and Lazarus, Pt. II. (Anæmia pseudoleukæmica infantum).

complete expulsion of the Bothriocephalus, the megaloblastic character of the blood formation quickly vanished,
was replaced by the normoblastic, and the patient rapidly
recovered. This observation is so unequivocal, that it
is a matter of surprise that Askanazy chooses to deduce
from it, the ready transition from megaloblasts to normoblasts; whereas it is clear and definite evidence that
megaloblasts are only produced under the influence of a specific intoxication. And in this way
the presence of megaloblasts in the pernicious anæmias
is to be explained. The megaloblastic degeneration of
the bone-marrow depends on the presence of certain
injurious influences, of which unfortunately we are as yet
ignorant. Were it possible to remove them, it is quite
certain à priori that the bone-marrow—if the disease
were not too advanced—would resume its normal normoblastic type of regeneration. Clinical observation supports
this contention in many cases. In megaloblastic anæmias
apparent cures are by no means rare, but sooner or later
a relapse occurs, and finally leads with certainty to a lethal
issue. These cases, familiar to every observer, prove with
certainty that the megaloblastic degeneration as such
may pass away, and that in isolated cases the conven-
tional treatment by arsenic suffices to bring about this
result. A definite cure however under these conditions
is not yet attained, since we do not know the ætiological
agent, still less can we remove it. For this reason,
the prognosis of megaloblastic anæmia, apart
from the group of Bothriocephalus anæmia, is
exceedingly bad.

# THE
# WHITE BLOOD CORPUSCLES.

# THE WHITE BLOOD CORPUSCLES.

THE physiological importance of the *white blood corpuscles* is so many sided that they form the most interesting chapter of the subject. That the white corpuscles play a significant part in the physiology and pathology of man has been recognised but slowly, obviously because there was at first some hesitancy in ascribing important functions to elements that are present in the blood in such relatively small numbers. A place in pathology was first assured to them by Virchow's discovery of leukæmia. The interest in the question was increased by Cohnheim's discovery that inflammation and suppuration are due to an emigration of the white blood corpuscles, and these conditions were particularly suitable for throwing light on normal processes. The fact that in diffuse inflammations, large quantities of pus are often produced in a short time, without the blood being thereby made poorer in leucocytes,—that the opposite indeed occurs,— necessitated the supposition that the source of the leucocytes must be extraordinarily productive. Hence in contradistinction to the red blood corpuscles, their small number is fully compensated by their exceptional power of regeneration.

Nevertheless, a considerable time elapsed before the

powerful impulse that started from Cohnheim, bore fruit
for clinical histology. As we have mentioned this was
due to the circumstance that an exact differentiation of
the various forms of leucocytes was very difficult with the
methods in use up to that time. Although such distinguished observers as Wharton Jones and Max Schultze
had been able to distinguish different types of leucocytes,
Cohnheim's work remained clinically fruitless since the
criteria they assigned were far too subtle for investigation
at the bedside. Virchow indeed, the discoverer of leucocytosis, interpreted it as an increase of the lymphocytes;
whereas it is chiefly produced by the polynuclear cells.
Only after the distinction was facilitated by the dry preparation and the use of stains, did interest in the white
corpuscles increase, and continue progressively to the
present day. This is borne out by the exceptionally exhaustive hæmatological literature, and particularly by that
of leucocytosis.

In spite of these advances, a retrograde movement in
the doctrine of the leucocytes has gained ground sur-
prisingly, especially in the last few years. Ever since
Virchow's description of the lymphocytes, observers have
tried to separate the various forms of leucocytes one from
another, and if possible to assign different places of origin
to these different kinds. There now suddenly appears an
endeavour to bring all the white blood corpuscles into
one class, and to regard the different forms as different
stages merely of the same kind of cells. The following
sections will shew that this tendency is unwarranted and
unpractical.

# I. NORMAL AND PATHOLOGICAL HISTOLOGY OF THE WHITE BLOOD CORPUSCLES.

THE classification of the white corpuscles of normal human blood, drawn up by Ehrlich, has been accepted by most authors, and we therefore give a short summary of it, as founded on the dry specimen.

1. The Lymphocytes. These are small cells, as a rule approximating in size to the red blood corpuscles. Their body is occupied by a large round homogeneously stained nucleus centrally situated, whilst the protoplasm surrounds the nucleus as a concentric border. Between nucleus and protoplasm there is often found a narrow areola, which doubtless results from artificial retraction. Nucleus and protoplasm are basophil, nevertheless in many methods of staining the protoplasm possesses a much stronger affinity for the basic stain than does the nucleus. The nucleus in these cases stands out as a bright spot from the deeply stained mass of protoplasm, which is reticulated in a peculiar manner.

Within the nucleus are often to be found one or two nucleoli with a relatively thick and deeply stained membrane. With methylene blue and similar dyes the protoplasm stains unequally, which is not to be considered as the expression of a granulation, as Ehrlich first assumed, but rather of a reticular structure. The contour of the lymphocytes is not quite smooth as a rule, at least in the larger forms, but is somewhat frayed, jagged, and uneven (Fig. 1). Small portions of the peripheral substance may repeatedly bud off, especially in the large forms, and circulate in the blood as free elements. In stained specimens, especially from lymphatic leukæmia, these forms, which completely resemble the protoplasm of the lymphocytes in their staining, may from their nature and origin be readily recognised.

As far as the further metamorphosis of the nucleus is concerned, a sharp notching of the border of the nucleus may occasionally be found, the further fate of which is shewn in the accompanying figure (Fig. 3). It is evident that in this case the resulting nuclear forms are quite different from those which are characteristic of the polynuclear elements.

The protoplasm possesses no special affinity for acid and neutral dyes, and hence in triacid and hæmatoxylin preparations the small lymphocytes are seen chiefly as lightly stained nuclei, apparently free. In the larger cells the protoplasm can be seen even in these preparations to be slightly stained. By the aid of the iodine-eosine method the reaction of the protoplasm of the lymphocytes is shewn to be strongly alkaline. They do not contain glycogen.

These properties taken as a whole constitute a picture completely characteristic of the lymphocytes; and these elements can thereby be diagnosed and separated from other forms, even when their size varies. Generally speaking, these cells, as above mentioned, are distinguished in the blood of the healthy adult by their small size, approximating to that of the red blood corpuscles.

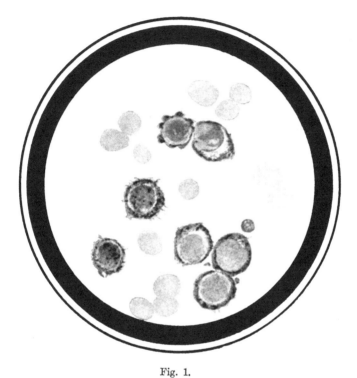

Fig. 1.

Fraying out of the protoplasmic border in large lymphocytes.   Free
plasma elements formed by budding.   ("Plasmolysis.")

(From a photograph of a preparation from chronic
lymphatic leukaemia.)

*To face page* 72

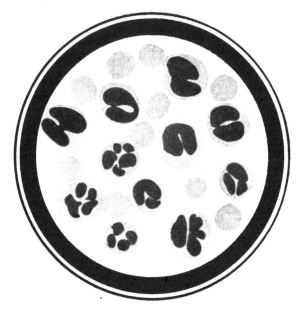

Fig 2.   (From Rieder's Atlas.)

Metamorphosis of the nucleus of the lymphocytes.

(Combined picture from a preparation from acute leukaemia.)

*To follow Fig.* 1

In the blood of children on the contrary larger forms are found even in health; and in lymphatic leukæmia particularly large forms occur, which are mistaken in various ways by unpractised observers. Thus Troje's "marrow cells" still figure in the literature, but have absolutely nothing to do with the marrow. They are large lymphocytes, as was established by A. Fränkel years afterwards.

In the normal blood of adults the number of the lymphocytes amounts to about 22—25 % of the colourless elements.

Increase of the lymphocytes alone occurs, but in comparison with that of the other forms, much more seldom, and will be conveniently called by the special names of "lymphocytosis" or "lymphæmia."

2. Sharply to be distinguished from the lymphocytes is the second group: the "large mononuclear leucocytes." These are large cells about twice to three times the size of the erythrocytes. They possess a large oval nucleus, as a rule eccentrically situated and staining feebly, and a relatively abundant protoplasm. The latter is free from granulations, feebly basophil, and in contrast to the protoplasm of the lymphocytes stains less deeply than the nucleus. This group is present in normal blood in but small numbers (about 1 %). They are separated from the lymphocytes because they are totally different in appearance, and because forms transitional between the two are not observed. It cannot yet be decided from which blood-producing organs these forms arise, whether from spleen or bone-marrow, although there are many reasons for regarding the latter as their place of origin.

These large mononuclear leucocytes change in the blood to the following kind:

3. "The transitional forms." These resemble the preceding, but are distinguished therefrom by deep notchings of the nucleus, which often give it an hour-glass shape, further by a somewhat greater affinity of the nucleus for stains, and by the presence of scanty neutrophil granulations in the protoplasm. The groups 2 and 3 comprise together about 2—4 % of the white blood corpuscles[1].

4. The (so-called) "polynuclear leucocytes." These arise in small part, as will be described later in detail, from the above-mentioned No. 3, within the blood stream. By far the larger part is produced fully formed in the bone-marrow, and emigrate to the blood. These cells are rather smaller than Nos. 3 and 2 and are distinguished by the following peculiarities: firstly by a peculiar polymorphous form of nucleus which gives the relatively long, irregularly bulged and indented nuclear rod the appearance of an S, Y, E or Z. The complete decomposition of this nuclear rod into three to four small round single nuclei may occur during life, as a natural process. Ehrlich first discovered it in a case of hæmorrhagic small, pox; it is frequently found in fresh exudations. Formerly when various reagents, for instance acetic acid, were customarily used, the decomposition of the nucleus into several parts was more frequently observed, and Ehrlich for this reason chose the not wholly appropriate name "polynuclear" for this form of cell. As this name has now been universally adopted, and misunderstandings cannot be expected, it is undoubtedly better to keep to it. The expression "Cells with polymorphous nuclei" would be more accurate.

[1] In enumerating the blood corpuscles, 2 and 3 may be counted separately or in one group.

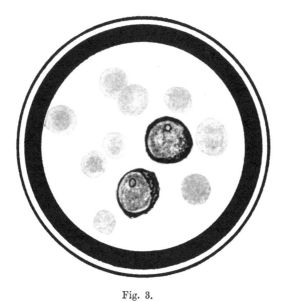

Fig. 3.

Nucleoli in larger lymphocytes.
(From a photograph of a preparation from chronic
lymphatic leukaemia.)

To face page 74

The nucleus stains very deeply with all dyes; the protoplasm possesses a strong attraction for most acid stains, and is unmistakeably characterised by the presence of a dense neutrophil granulation. The reaction of the protoplasm is alkaline, to a less degree however than in the lymphocytes. No free glycogen is contained in the polynuclear cells as a rule; nevertheless in certain diseases cells are always found which give a marked iodine reaction. In this manner the appearance of cells containing glycogen in diabetes was first proved. (Ehrlich, Gabritschewsky, Livierato.) The iodine reaction in the white blood corpuscles is also seen in severe contusions and fractures, in pneumonias, in rapidly progressing phlegmata from streptococcus and staphylococcus, after protracted narcosis (Goldberger and Weiss).

Ehrlich explains the appearance of glycogen as follows. The glycogen is not present in the cell as such, but in the form of a compound, which does not stain with iodine. This compound readily splits off glycogen, which then gives the iodine reaction[1].

We cannot regard the perinuclear green granules, described by Neusser in the polynuclear cells, as pre-existing. (See p. 42.)

The number of polynuclear leucocytes in the blood of the healthy adult amounts to about $70-72\,^{\circ}/_{\circ}$ of the total white corpuscles. (Einhorn.)[2]

---

[1] The assumption of Czerny, that the cells which react to iodine emigrate from suppurating foci, is without foundation. A simple investigation of freshly inflamed tissue is sufficient to show that the cells which have wandered from the blood stream soon contain glycogen.

[2] Kanthack described this group as "finely granular oxyphil" cells. Their granules stain red in eosine and in eosine-methylene blue solutions, but the colour is different from that of the true eosinophil cells, and much less intense. In the latter mixture they stain really with the methylene blue salt of eosine. Their true nature is shown by their behaviour with the triacid solution.

5. The eosinophil cells. These are characterised by a coarse, round granulation, staining deeply with acid dyes, and similar in other respects to the polynuclear neutrophils. With faint staining, a thin peripheral layer of the eosinophil granule is seen more deeply stained than the interior. The nucleus as a rule is not so deeply stained as in the polynuclear neutrophil, but otherwise in its general shape is completely similar. Both forms have in common a considerable contractility, which renders possible their emigration from the vessels, and their appearance in exudations and in pus. The size of the eosinophils frequently exceeds that of the neutrophils. Their number is normally about 2—4 % of the white cells.

6. The mast cells. These are present, though very sparingly, in every normal blood; 0·5 % is their maximum number in health.

Their intensely basophil granulation, of very irregular size and unequal distribution, must specially be mentioned. The granulation possesses the further peculiarity, in that with the majority of basic dyes it stains, not in the pure colour of the dye, but metachromatically—most deeply with thionin. As Dr Morgenroth found, the deviation from the colour of the dye is still more marked with Kresyl-violet-R (Mülheim manufactory), when the granules stain almost a pure brown.

The staining power of the nuclei is very small, and it is therefore hard to make out the shape of the nucleus without the use of difficult methods. In triacid preparations the granulation is unstained, and the mast cells appear as clear, polynuclear cells, free from granules.

---

So much for the colourless cells in the blood of the normal adult.

In pathological cases, not only do the forms so far mentioned occur in altered numbers, but abnormal cells also make their appearance. To these belong:

1. **Mononuclear cells with neutrophil granulation.** ("Myelocytes," Ehrlich.) Generally they are bulky, with a relatively large, faintly staining nucleus, often fairly centrally placed, and equally surrounded by protoplasm on all sides. A fundamental distinction from the large mononuclear cells lies in the fact that the protoplasm exhibits a more or less numerous neutrophil granulation. Besides the larger myelocytes, much smaller forms, approximating to the size of the erythrocytes are also found. All transitions between these two stages are likewise met with. In contradistinction to the polynuclear neutrophil elements, these mononuclear forms shew no amœboid movement on the warm stage. They form a constant characteristic of myelogenic leukæmia, and in these cases generally occur in large numbers.

Reinbach has found them in a case of lympho-sarcoma with metastases in the bone-marrow. A. Lazarus observed their transitory occurrence in moderate number in a severe posthæmorrhagic anæmia. M. Beck observed them in the blood of a patient with severe mercury poisoning. They are also frequently found in children's diseases, especially in *anæmia pseudoleukœmica infantum*. K. Elze established their presence in a boy of 15 months, suffering from a slowly progressing tuberculosis of the lymphatic glands.

The appearance of myelocytes in infectious diseases is particularly interesting. Rieder had previously demonstrated that myelocytes may be present in acute inflammatory leucocytoses; and recently a thorough work by C. S. Engel has appeared upon the occurrence of myelocytes in diphtheria. Engel discovered the interesting fact, that myelocytes are often to be found in children suffering from diphtheria, and further made the important observation that a high percentage of myelocytes ($3\cdot6$—$16\cdot4\,^0/_0$ of the white elements) only occurs in severe cases, and points to an unfavourable prognosis. Myelocytes are also present in mild cases, though not constantly and in much smaller number. Türk has recently undertaken a very exact and thorough analysis of their occurrence in infectious diseases, in the course of which he accurately tabulated the white corpuscles in a large number of cases. The results he obtained in pneumonia are especially characteristic, for he found at the commencement of the disease that myelocytes are not seen at all or only very scantily : and it is only at the time of the crisis, or directly afterwards, that they become specially numerous. In isolated cases the increase at this time was very considerable ; and in one case amounted almost to $12\,^0/_0$ of all neutrophil cells.

2. Mononuclear eosinophil cells ("eosinophil myelocytes"). H. F. Müller was the first to point out their importance. They constitute the eosinophil analogue of the previous group, and are much larger than the polynuclear eosinophils ; medium and small sized examples are often found in leukæmia. Eosinophil myelocytes are almost constantly present in myelogenous leukæmia and in anæmia pseudolymphatica infantum. Apart from these two diseases they are very rarely found ; Mendel saw them for example in a case of myxœdema, Türk quite exceptionally in some infectious diseases.

3. Small neutrophil pseudo lymphocytes. They

are about as large as the small lymphocytes, possess a rounded deeply stained nucleus, and a small shell of protoplasm studded with a neutrophil granulation. The relatively deep stain of the nucleus and the small share of the protoplasm in the total cell body prevent confusion with the small forms of myelocytes, which never reach such small dimensions. The neutrophil pseudolymphocytes are exceedingly infrequent, and represent products of division of the polynuclear cells; they were first described by Ehrlich in a case of hæmorrhagic small-pox. The process of division goes on in the blood in such a manner that the nuclear rod first divides into two to four single nuclei, and then the whole cell splits up into as many fragments. These cells occur also in fresh pleuritic exudations. After a time the nucleus of these cells becomes free, and the little masses of protoplasm thus cut off are taken up mostly by the spleen substance. The free nucleus likewise shares in the destruction. It is of the greatest importance that these cells, which up to the present have not elsewhere been described, should receive more attention. They must be of significance, in particular for the question of transitory hyperleucocytosis, which is by some referred to a destruction, by others to an altered localisation of the white blood corpuscles.

4. "Stimulation forms" were first described by Türk, and are mononuclear non-granulated cells. They possess a protoplasm staining with various degrees of intensity, but in any case giving with triacid solution an extraordinarily deep dark-brown, and further a round simple nucleus often eccentrically situated, stained a moderately deep bluish-green, with however a distinct chromatin network. The smallest forms stand between

the lymphocytes and the large mononuclear leucocytes, but approach the first named as a whole in their size and general appearance. According to Türk's investigations, these cells often occur simultaneously with, and under the same conditions as the myelocytes. Their importance cannot at present be accurately gauged. Possibly they form an early stage of development of the nucleated red blood corpuscles, as the deeply staining and homogeneous protoplasm seems to indicate.

With the description of these abnormal forms of white corpuscles all occurring forms are by no means exhausted. We are here excepting completely the variations in size which particularly affect the polynuclear and eosinophil cells, and which lead to dwarf and giant forms of them. For however considerable the difference in size, these cells always possess characteristics sufficient for an exact diagnosis. But besides these, isolated cells of an especially large kind are found—particularly in leukæmic blood, and concerning their importance and relationship we are up to the present in the dark.

## II. ON THE PLACES OF ORIGIN OF THE
## WHITE BLOOD CORPUSCLES.

FOR the comprehension of the histology of the blood
as a whole, it is of great importance to obtain an exact
knowledge how and to what extent the three organs,
which are undoubtedly very closely connected with
the blood, lymphatic glands, bone-marrow, and spleen,
contribute to its formation. The most direct way of
deciding the question experimentally by excision of the
organs in question, is unfortunately only available for the
spleen. The part played by the lymphatic glands and
bone-marrow, whose exclusion *in toto* is not possible,
must mainly be determined by anatomical and clinical
considerations. But only by a careful combination of
experiments on animals, of anatomical investigations,
and especially, of clinical observations on a large scale,
can light be thrown on these very difficult questions.
It cannot be emphasised sufficiently how important it
is that everyone engaging in hæmatological work should
first of all collect a large series of general observations;
otherwise errors are bound to occur. For instance, the
endeavour is often made to compensate the lack of
personal experience by careful literary studies; but in
this way the histology of the blood falls into a vicious

circle, of which the new phase of blood histology affords many examples. And it is characteristic of this kind of work that from the investigation of a single rare case, most far-reaching conclusions on the general pathology of the blood are at once drawn; *e.g.* Troje's paper, in which having failed to recognise the lymphocytic character of a case of leukæmia, and believing therefore that he had to do with a myelogenous leukæmia, the author denied and completely reversed all that had been previously established about this disease. It is equally hard to avoid errors if one confines oneself exclusively to animal experiments, without supplementing these by clinical experience, as is shewn by the numerous papers of Uskoff. Not the anatomist, not the physiologist, but only the clinician is in the position to discuss these problems.

In the introduction to this chapter we have already alluded to the striking retrograde movement in hæmatology at the present time, brought about by the view that the white corpuscles as a whole are derived from the lymphocytes. If we disregard the embryological investigations on this point (Saxer), anatomists, physiologists, and clinicians alike have taken up a similar point of view. Among anatomical papers we may refer to those of Gulland, according to whom all varieties of leucocytes are but different stages of development of one and the same element. He distinguishes hyaline, acidophil and basophil cells, and derives all from the lymphocytes. Arnold advocates similar views, though in a negative form. He says that a distinction between so-called lymphocytes and the leucocytes with polymorphous nuclei, on the grounds of the form of the cell and nature of the nucleus, is not possible at the present time. Neither is a classification based on the granules admissible, since the same granules occur in different cells, and different granules in the same cell. The work of Gulland and Arnold takes into consideration the differential staining of the granules in various ways. In spite of their facts we disagree with their conclusions; and we shall therefore have to analyse them in the special description of the granulated cells and granules.

Recently (since 1889) Uskoff has in particular published experimental work in this province of hæmatology. This has led him to see in the white blood corpuscles the developmental series of one kind of cell, and to distinguish in it, three stages: (1) "young cells," which correspond to our lymphocytes; (2) "ripe cells" (globules mûrs), large cells with fairly large and irregularly shaped nucleus, which are therefore our large mononuclear and transitional forms; (3) "old cells" (globules vieux), which represent our polynuclear cells. The eosinophil cells are completely excluded from this classification. Amongst clinicians A. Fränkel has recently gone in the same direction, and on the grounds of his experience in acute leukæmias has supported the view of Uskoff, that the lymphocytes are to be regarded as young cells, and early stages of the other leucocytes. But few authors (for instance C. S. Engel, Ribbert) have raised a protest to this mixing of all cell forms of the blood, and have held to the old classification of Ehrlich. But as it is emphatically taught in numerous medical works that all these cells are closely related, the grounds for sharply separating the lymphocytes from the bone-marrow group may here be shortly summarised, and stress laid on the great importance which this apparently purely theoretical question has for clinical observation. We shall come to most important conclusions upon this point when we consider more closely the share which the various regions of the hæmatopoietic system take in the formation of the blood, and especially of the colourless elements.

## α. **The Spleen.**

The question whether the **spleen** produces white blood corpuscles has played a large part from the earliest times of hæmatology.

Endeavours were first made to investigate the participation of the spleen in the formation of the white blood corpuscles by counting the white corpuscles in the afferent and efferent vessels of the spleen. It was thought that the blood-forming power of the spleen was proved by the larger number of corpuscles in the vein as compared with the artery. The results of these enumerations however are very varying; the investigators who found a relative increase in the vein are opposed by other investigators equally reliable; and with the experience of the present day one would not lay any value on these experiments.

We must emphasise the fact, established by later researches, that after extirpation of the spleen, an enlargement of various lymphatic glands occurs. The alterations of the thyroid, which have been observed by many authors, cannot be described as constant.

Further, the blood investigations which Mosler, Robin, Winogradow, Zersas and others have carried on in animals and man after removal of the spleen must here be mentioned. These have already proved that a leucocytosis occurs after some considerable time. Prof. Kurloff carried out detailed investigations in 1888 in Ehrlich's laboratory, and carefully studied the condition of the blood after extirpation of the spleen. As the work of Prof. Kurloff has so far only appeared in Russian, his important results may be here recorded more fully. For his researches, Kurloff employed the guinea-pig, as this animal by its peculiar blood is specially suited for this purpose.

In order to give a systematic account of the results of these important investigations, we must first shortly sketch the normal histology of the blood of the guinea-pig according to Kurloff.

In the blood of the healthy guinea-pig the following elements are found.

## I. Cells bearing granules.

1. Polynuclear, with pseudoeosinophil granulation. This granulation, which Ehrlich had previously found in the rabbit, is easily distinguishable from the true eosinophil, since it is much finer, and stains quite differently in eosine-aurantia-nigrosin mixtures. One principal distinction between these two forms of cells lies in the fact that, according to Kurloff, this granulation is very easily dissolved by acid, but remains unchanged in alkaline solutions; doubtless an indication that the granulation consists of a basic body soluble with difficulty, which with acids forms soluble salts. The true eosinophil granulation remains, on the other hand, quite unchanged under these conditions.

These pseudoeosinophil, polynuclear cells, correspond functionally to the neutrophil polynuclear of man; their number amounts to 40—50 % of the total white cells. The red bone-marrow is to be regarded as the place of origin of this kind of cell. It contains very many pseudoeosinophil cells, and indeed all stages are to be found in it, from the mononuclear cells bearing granules to the fully formed polynuclear.

2. The typical eosinophil leucocytes, which fully correspond to those found in man, and amount to about 10 % of the number of the white.

3. The "nigrosinophil cells," as they are called by Kurloff. In their general appearance, in the size of the cell and the granulation, they completely correspond to the eosinophil cell. The only distinction between them consists in a chemical difference in the granulation. These cells stain in the colour of nigrosin in the aurantia-eosin-nigrosin mixture, whilst the eosinophil cells become red. The two granulations always shew different shades in the triacid preparation as well; for the nigrosinophil cells stain a blacker hue.

## II. Cells free from granules.

### (a) Cells with vacuoles.

This is a quite peculiar group, characteristic for the blood of the guinea-pig. It shews transitions in the blood, from large mononuclear to transitional and polynuclear forms, but is marked by the lack of any kind of granulation. Instead of the latter, we find in these cells a roundish, nucleus-like form in the protoplasm, which also takes the nuclear stains, and possibly is to be considered an accessory nucleus. We have received the impression that we have here to deal with a vacuole filled with substance secreted by the cell. In a large series of preparations, it is possible to obtain some elucidation of the development and fate of these appearances. They first appear as point-like granules in the protoplasm, bearing no relation to the cell nucleus; they gradually increase, and acquire a considerable circumference. When they have attained about the size of the cell nucleus, they, or rather their contents, appear to break through the protoplasmic membrane and to leave the cell.

The number of the vacuole containing cells is 15—20 °/₀ of the colourless blood corpuscles.

### (β) Typical lymphocytes.

Their appearance completely corresponds with that of human lymphocytes as described above. They make up 30—35 °/₀ of the total number of leucocytes.

Now Kurloff in the course of extremely careful and laborious researches, estimated the total number of leucocytes, and then from the percentage numbers, the total quantity of pseudoeosinophil, neutrophil, eosinophil, vacuole containing cells, and lymphocytes, and could thus demonstrate that in uncomplicated cases of removal of the spleen, where inflammatory processes, accompanied by an increase of the polynuclear neutrophil corpuscles, were avoided, a gradual increase of the lymphocytes alone in course of time results. This may be a two- or threefold increase, whereas the numbers of all other elements remain unchanged.

Kurloff obtained his figures as follows : first he estimated the relative proportion of the different kinds of white blood corpuscles one to another in a large number of cells (500 to 1000). A count of this kind however gives no evidence as to whether one or other kind of cell is absolutely increased or diminished. A fall in the percentage of the lymph cells may be brought about by two quite different factors: (1) by a diminished production of lymphocytes, (2) by an increased influx of polynuclear forms, which naturally lowers the relative count of the lymphocytes. It was therefore necessary to obtain a method which would shew alterations in the absolute number of the individual forms of leucocytes. Kurloff used for this purpose the "comparative field"; that is, he counted by the aid of a moveable stage the different forms which lay on a definite area (22 sq. mm.) of the dried blood preparation. This procedure gave very exact results, as only faultlessly prepared, and regularly spread preparations were used. The following figures (from Exp. II.) illustrate the method and its results:

| April 12 | 52 % pseudo-eos. | 10 % lymphocytes counted. |
| Sept. 2 (one month after the operation) | 22 % ,, | 53 % ,, ,, |

By the aid of the comparative surface, these figures

were supplemented by the following averages. On each surface used for comparison were found:

April 12   38 white = 19·8 pseudo-eos.   10·6 lymphocytes.
Sept. 2    81   ,,     18·0      ,,       46·9       ,,

From this example it follows without doubt, that the total number of the white blood corpuscles had about doubled itself, but that in this increase the lymphocytes exclusively were concerned, and the pseudo-eosinophil cells had not undergone the smallest increase.

The results which Kurloff obtained by means of this method in animals whose spleens had been removed, may be illustrated by one of his original researches and its accompanying chart and table.

Exp. I. Young female, weight 234 gr. Number of red corpuscles in a cubic millimeter of blood 5,780,000. Number of white 10,700. On April 19, 1888, the spleen was removed, the wound healed by first intention. The results of the further investigation of the blood are found in the following table.

From the chart and table, the number on the surface of comparison of the white blood corpuscles is seen to have more than doubled itself in the first seven months, and that this increase was solely dependent on the flooding of the blood by lymphocytes. The nucleated or bone-marrow elements and the large mononuclear cells remained continuously at the same level during the whole period. The changes in the percentage proportions ran somewhat differently. The percentages rose from 35 to 66 % for the lymphocytes only, whilst for the other forms they distinctly fell: for the nucleated from 44 % to 22 % and for the large mononuclear from 18 % to 9 %. It was only in the course of the second year that a very considerable relative and absolute increase of the eosinophil cells appeared: the values rose gradually from about 1·0 % to 28·9 % or from 0·5 to 13·9 on each comparison area. The last examination of the blood in this animal was made on April 30, 1890, that is, two years after the removal of the spleen. The animal was quite healthy, bore four healthy young guinea-pigs by a father whose spleen had been

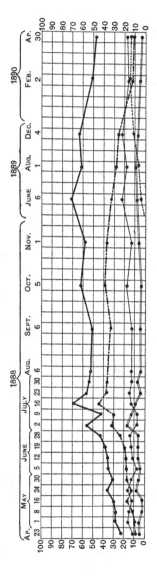

CHART TO EXPT. No. I. (cp. Table, page 89. The figures in the chart refer to comparative surfaces.)

Thick line—total number of leucocytes

Thin line—number of nucleated, pseudo-
    eosinophil cells

Broken line—lymphocytes

Double line—large mononuclear cells

Dotted line—eosinophil cells

removed. The young have a completely normal spleen, and their blood likewise shows no abnormalities.

## TABLE I.

| Date | Leucocytes | | Pseudo-eosinophil cells | | Lympho-cytes | | Large mono-nuclear cells | | Eosinophil cells | | Nigro-sinophil cells | |
|---|---|---|---|---|---|---|---|---|---|---|---|---|
| | Total | On comparative surface | % | On comparative surface | % | On comparative surface | % | On comparative surface | % | On comparative surface | % | On comparative surface |
| **1888** | | | | | | | | | | | | |
| April 19 | 500 | — | 44·7 | — | 35·4 | — | 18·4 | — | 1·1 | — | 0·5 | — |
| 23 | 990 | 24 | 40·4 | 9·7 | 35·6 | 8·5 | 21·6 | 5·2 | 1·9 | 0·4 | 0·4 | 0·09 |
| May 1 | 858 | 28 | 47·0 | 13·6 | 32·6 | 9·1 | 18·0 | 5·0 | 0·9 | 0·2 | 0·3 | 0·08 |
| 8 | 934 | 28 | 45·2 | 12·6 | 40·3 | 11·3 | 14·3 | 4·0 | 0·6 | 0·2 | 0·4 | 0·1 |
| 16 | 1122 | 30 | 38·4 | 11·5 | 47·7 | 14·3 | 10·3 | 3·1 | 3·3 | 0·9 | 0·2 | 0·06 |
| 24 | 1722 | 35 | 40·1 | 14·0 | 35·0 | 12·2 | 23·6 | 8·3 | 1·0 | 0·3 | 0·1 | 0·03 |
| 30 | 900 | 30 | 36·6 | 10·9 | 44·4 | 13·3 | 18·4 | 5·5 | 0·1 | 0·03 | 0·3 | 0·09 |
| June 5 | 825 | 33 | 28·4 | 9·4 | 49·3 | 16·2 | 20·0 | 6·6 | 1·7 | 0·6 | 0·4 | 0·1 |
| 12 | 1314 | 33 | 28·0 | 9·3 | 49·0 | 16·2 | 20·0 | 6·6 | 2·2 | 0·7 | 0·8 | 0·3 |
| 19 | 917 | 37 | 32·4 | 11·9 | 52·3 | 19·3 | 14·5 | 5·4 | 0·6 | 0·3 | 0·2 | 0·07 |
| 28 | 802 | 42 | 30·5 | 12·8 | 56·4 | 23·7 | 11·7 | 4·9 | 0·7 | 0·3 | 0·4 | 0·2 |
| July 2 | 1062 | 56 | 16·5 | 9·2 | **57·1** | **31·9** | 25·6 | 10·3 | 1·2 | 0·7 | 1·2 | 0·7 |
| 9 | 1245 | 51 | 17·6 | 8·9 | **59·1** | **30·1** | 21·8 | 11·1 | 0·8 | 0·4 | 0·8 | 0·4 |
| 16 | 974 | 69 | 17·5 | 12·0 | **66·4** | **45·8** | 15·7 | 10·8 | 0·2 | 0·1 | 0·2 | 0·1 |
| 23 | 1156 | 58 | 21·7 | 12·6 | **67·2** | **38·9** | 9·5 | 5·5 | 1·5 | 0·9 | 0·2 | 0·1 |
| 30 | 802 | 54 | 20·2 | 10·7 | **65·4** | **34·6** | 12·8 | 6·8 | 1·4 | 0·7 | — | — |
| Aug. 6 | 910 | 52 | 21·7 | 11·3 | **67·3** | **34·9** | 9·7 | 4·9 | 1·0 | 0·5 | 0·3 | 0·2 |
| Sept. 6 | 815 | 51 | 23·0 | 11·7 | **65·3** | **33·5** | 9·8 | 4·9 | 0·9 | 0·5 | 0·4 | 0·2 |
| Oct. 5 | 625 | 62 | 26·4 | 16·3 | **64·4** | **39·9** | 8·5 | 5·2 | 0·6 | 0·4 | — | — |
| Nov. 4 | 800 | 58 | 22·5 | 13·0 | **66·4** | **38·5** | 9·6 | 7·3 | 0·9 | 0·5 | 0·5 | 0·2 |
| **1889** | | | | | | | | | | | | |
| April 10 | 700 | — | 29·8 | — | 53·3 | — | 14·8 | — | 1·2 | — | 0·6 | — |
| June 6 | 900 | 71 | 28·2 | 20·0 | 50·1 | 35·6 | 12·9 | 9·1 | **8·2** | **5·8** | 0·6 | 0·4 |
| Aug. 1 | 670 | 62 | 30·6 | 18·9 | 44·2 | 27·4 | 15·2 | 9·4 | **9·6** | **5·9** | 0·4 | 0·2 |
| Dec. 4 | 731 | 63 | 36·0 | 22·0 | 38·3 | 24·1 | 11·3 | 7·1 | **13·3** | **8·7** | 0·6 | 0·4 |
| **1890** | | | | | | | | | | | | |
| Feb. 2 | 622 | 51 | 32·3 | 16·5 | 30·1 | 15·3 | 11·1 | 5·6 | **26·0** | **13·2** | 0·5 | 0·2 |
| April 30 | 500 | 48 | 36·5 | 17·5 | 24·5 | 11·7 | 9·4 | 4·5 | **28·9** | **13·9** | 0·6 | 0·3 |

The results of further investigations, which we here shortly repeat in tabular form, shew that in this experiment No. I. we are not dealing with an abnormal phenomenon of an exceptional animal.

| No. of Expt. | Number of white blood corpuscles | | |
|---|---|---|---|
| | Before the splenectomy | At the end of the first year | At the end of the second year |
| 1 | 10,700 | 14,200 | 18,000 |
| 2 | 12,000 | 27,600 | 32,000 |
| 4 | 15,000 | 19,200 | 19,000 |
| Average | 12,600 | 20,333 | 23,300 |

By estimating the percentage proportion of the single kinds of white corpuscles, Kurloff obtained the following result:

| No. of the Experiment | Before the operation | | | | At the end of the first year | | | | At the end of the second year | | | |
|---|---|---|---|---|---|---|---|---|---|---|---|---|
| | Polynuclear granular cells | Lymphocytes | Mononuclear | Eosinophil | Polynuclear granular cells | Lymphocytes | Mononuclear | Eosinophil | Polynuclear granular cells | Lymphocytes | Mononuclear | Eosinophil |
| 1 | 4782 | 3788 | 1969 | 117 | 4232 | 1568 | 2101 | 170 | 6570 | 4410 | 1692 | 5202 |
| 2 | 6276 | 3360 | 2244 | 72 | 5464 | 16615 | 2980 | 2539 | 5824 | 20861 | 2688 | 2240 |
| 4 | 6715 | 5250 | 2595 | 450 | 6568 | 10041 | 3686 | 96 | 7108 | 3009 | 2138 | 7543 |

From these researches we draw the following conclusions.

1. The spleen is not an indispensable, vitally important organ for the guinea-pig, since that animal bears splenectomy without loss of health, developes normally, and gains well in weight.

2. The hypertrophy and hyperplasia of the lymph

glands, particularly of the mesenteric glands, which develop after the operation correspond to a lymphocytosis, which makes its appearance in the course of the first year after the operation so constantly that it may be looked upon as a characteristic sign of the absence of the spleen. This increase may amount to double and more. We must therefore assume that the deficiency of splenic function may be met by the lymphatic glandular system. This period of lymphæmia may doubtless in some animals persist for years in exceptional cases; in the majority, however, the lymphæmia diminishes in the course of the first year, and indeed subnormal quantities of lymphocytes may then be produced.

3. The cells of the bone-marrow, on the contrary, and the polynuclear pseudoeosinophil cells do not show the least variation in the course of the first year. Bearing in mind that under normal conditions these cells are met with exclusively in the bone-marrow, and that inflammation in animals after removal of the spleen is accompanied by an acute pseudoeosinophil leucocytosis, exactly as in normal animals, one must admit that the production and function of this kind of cell are quite independent of the spleen. Hence there can be no doubt about their myelogenic nature.

4. It is especially important that the mononuclear and the leucocytes associated with them, undergo no increase. As these cells under normal circumstances occur both in the spleen and in the bone-marrow, we must assume that normally also the bone-marrow is responsible for the majority of this kind in the blood, and that the deficiency in the splenic contribution can be easily covered by a slightly raised activity of the bone-marrow. Were the share of the spleen important,

from general biological considerations, an over-production of the kind of cell in question must occur in the vicarious organs.

5. The increase of the eosinophil cells, which constantly makes its appearance in the second year after the operation, is highly interesting, and leads to a really enormous rise in their absolute and relative numbers. Their percentage number once rose to 34·6 %, and their absolute quantity amounted at the end of the second year on the average to 30—50-fold their original number (see table).

Hence it follows from Kurloff's researches that the spleen of the guinea-pig plays quite an unimportant part in the formation of the white blood corpuscles, and that after splenectomy in the first year compensation occurs only in the lymph-glands, followed in the second year by a great increase of the eosinophil cells. It is to be particularly insisted once again that the spleen has nothing at all to do with the formation of the pseudoeosinophil polynuclear cells, which are the analogues of the polynuclear neutrophils of man.

How do observations on man stand in the light of Kurloff's observations, which might be regarded as depending on peculiarities of the particular kind of animal ?

Completely analogous material is afforded by cases, in which in healthy people a splenectomy has been necessary in consequence of trauma. Unfortunately the material available for this purpose is extremely rare ; and it would be of the utmost value if the alterations of the blood in such a case were systematically studied for a period of years. We have ourselves begun our observations in two patients directly after the operation, but were unable to continue them, as death occurred within the first week after the extirpation. Up to the present only seven cases of rupture of the spleen with subsequent splenectomy have been published, as is stated in the collection of cases of v. Beck. In two only, of these seven cases, one of Riequer's (Breslau) the other of v. Beck's (Karlsruhe) was a cure effected. Through the courtesy of the above-mentioned gentlemen, we were able to investigate speci-mens from these two patients.

In the case of v. Beck the operation was performed on June 15, 1897. We received a dry blood preparation about 6 months after operation. Investigation showed a considerable lymphæmia : the bulk of the lymphocytes belonged to the larger kinds : the eosinophil cells were certainly not increased. For other reasons an exact numerical analysis could not be undertaken. We hope to be able to follow the further course of this case.

In the second case the operation was performed on May 17, 1892, by Dr Riequer of Breslau, for trauma, and later described. We made counts in oldish and fresh preparations. It is worthy of notice that this case is not uncomplicated, as an amputation of the thigh was performed shortly after the splenectomy on account of gangrene.

We found the following figures.

| Preparations from | Polynuclear | Lympho-cytes | Eosinophil | Large mononuclear |
|---|---|---|---|---|
| June 12, 1892 | 81·9 % | 15·9 % | 1·3 % | — |
| October 11, 1892 | 80·0 % | 13·7 % | 4·0 % | 1·7 % |
| September, 1897 | 56·8 % | 33·1 % | 3·5 % | 1·5 % |

It is much to be regretted that dry preparations only at the beginning and at the end of the five year period of observation were at our disposal. It appears from the paper of Riequer as if in this case the lymphocytosis had established itself one month after the operation, and had lasted for a very long time, just as Kurloff has found in some animal experiments. Just as little as a polynuclear increase is abnormal, is an increase of the lymphocytes remarkable; and in this case the lymphocytic increase was recognisable after the end of the fifth year. The eosinophil cells oscillate at this period about the upper normal limit. From all that we know, it is probable that their number in the meantime had undergone an intercurrent increase.

The cases are more frequent in which a splenectomy has been undertaken on account of disease of the spleen. Amongst these, the clearest results are à priori to be expected from splenic cysts, since the part of the spleen not affected by the cyst formation often shews quite a normal structure, and therefore is physiologically active. On the other hand, the excision of chronic splenic tumours may be—for the blood condition—of no importance inasmuch as the function of the spleen may have previously long been eliminated by pathological changes.

Amongst these cases, we must in the first place mention the well-known and carefully investigated case of B. Credé. In a man 44 years of age the spleen was extirpated on account of a large splenic cyst. Within two months of the operation there developed a thoroughly leukæmic condition of the blood, exclusively brought about by the increase of the lymphocytes, as is seen from the results of Credé and the table contained in his paper. It is further remarkable that four weeks after the operation a painful doughy swelling of the whole thyroid appeared, which remained, with variations, for nearly four months. With the general recovery of the patient this shrank to a small remnant. We notice further that this very interesting swelling of the thyroid, which doubtless stands in the closest connection with the splenectomy, is nevertheless no constant accompaniment of this operation, as for instance in the case of v. Beck, where it was not present.

The most recent work on extirpation of the spleen for tumours is from Hartmann and Vasquez. As the result of their researches the authors arrive at the following conclusions:

1. A slight post-operative increase of the red blood corpuscles and a true acute hyperleucocytosis occur and pass rapidly away.

2. The hæmoglobin equivalent of the corpuscles sinks at first but recovers its original value by degrees.

3. 4—8 weeks afterwards a lymphocytosis of varying duration is established.

4. Later, after many months, a moderate eosinophilia occurs.

We have ourselves been able to investigate three conclusive cases.

The first was a patient, which we were ourselves enabled to investigate by the courtesy of Dr A. Neumann. The patient's spleen was removed by E. Hahn on account of an echinococcus on Feb. 5, 1895. One may well assume that before the operation the spleen no longer discharged its normal function. On Sept. 2, 1897, we found the following numerical proportions:

| | |
|---|---|
| Polynuclear neutrophil | 76·5 %, |
| Lymphocytes | 18·4 %, |
| Eosinophil | 3·4 %, |
| Large mononuclear | 1·1 %, |
| Mast cells | 0·4 %. |

A condition therefore which was quite normal. In this connection it must be mentioned that an incipient phthisis pulmonum existed at the time, to which we must attribute an increase of the polynuclear elements, and without which the percentage figures of the lymphocytes and eosinophils would perhaps have been greater.

For the knowledge of the two other cases we are indebted to the kindness of Professor Jounescu of Bucharest. The one case was of a man of about 40 years of age, in whom splenectomy was undertaken on Sept. 27, 1897, for an enlarged spleen. Healing by first intention. The white blood corpuscles were permanently increased. The proportion of white to red was 1 : 120 to 1 : 130, the average number of red was 3,000,000. Our own examination of preparations obtained some two months after the operation, shewed a distinct lymphæmia, and also a preponderance of the larger lymph cells. The eosinophil and mast cells were plainly increased. We are unable to give more exact numerical data, as the preparations sent to us were not spread with sufficient regularity.

From the second case, which was also operated upon for enlargement of the spleen, we unfortunately only obtained much damaged preparations. Nevertheless so much could with certainty be established—that there was no considerable increase of the lymphocytes. The eosinophils on the contrary were increased distinctly, the mast cells to a lesser extent. It is probable that the increase of both of the latter kinds of cell was not a consequence of the extirpation of the spleen alone, but rather the expression of the reactive changes, which had already begun before the operation, from the exclusion of the splenic function.

Cases of splenectomy of this kind are transitional to the chronic diseases of the spleen. The latter present great difficulties, for one never knows how far in the most chronic diseases the other organs are damaged or influenced by the general illness.

An increase of the lymphocytes, so long as an affection of the lymphatic glands may be excluded, should be referred to functional exclusion of the spleen.

On the other hand, an increase of eosinophil cells associated with a chronic tumour of the spleen, is analogous to Kurloff's secondary reaction of the bone-

marrow. Such cases are frequently found in the literature. For instance Müller and Rieder bring forward
three cases of splenic tumour caused by congenital syphilis,
cirrhosis of the liver, neoplasm in the cranial cavity, and
in which the numbers of the eosinophils amounted to
$12.3\%$, $7.0\%$, $6.5\%$ respectively. In three cases of acute
splenic tumour in typhoid fever the figure $0.31\%$ with
a maximum of $0.82\%$, was found. These authors have
already raised the question "whether the increase of the
eosinophil cells is connected with the splenic tumour or
the bone-marrow? Perhaps the functional activity of
the latter is vicariously raised to meet the more or less
complete exclusion of the spleen from the formation of
the blood; since Ehrlich has distinctly asserted that the
probable place of formation of the eosinophil cells is
the bone-marrow."

From what has been brought forward no doubt can
now remain that the question has been decided quite in
Ehrlich's favour.

But what then are the physiological functions of the
spleen, since that organ is unnecessary for the persistence
of life? Doubtless its chief duty is the taking up of the
greater part of the decaying fragments of red and white
blood corpuscles in the blood-stream, so that this valuable
material is not quite lost for the organism. Thus Ponfick
has found that after destruction of the red corpuscles
the spleen takes up a portion of their "shadows," and
for this reason calls the splenic tumour a spodogenous
splenic tumour (σπόδος, ruins). Ehrlich has made a corresponding observation for the products of dissolution
of the white blood corpuscles, and has proved that the
splenic tumour which occurs in many infectious diseases
and in phosphorus poisoning is to a large extent caused

by the parenchyma of the spleen taking up the remains of the neutrophil protoplasm.

The question of the relation of the spleen to the fresh formation of red blood corpuscles is a problem of comparative anatomy. Observations on this point made on one kind of animal can certainly not claim validity for other kinds. In lower vertebrates, as in fishes, frogs, tortoises, and also in birds, the blood-forming activity of the spleen is pronounced and of great importance. In mammalia on the other hand, in some cases this function cannot be demonstrated, and in others only to a very small degree. In the spleen of normal mice nucleated red blood corpuscles are seen in relatively large numbers; in the rabbit they are less numerous and often only to be found with difficulty. In the dog they only make their appearance after anæmia from loss of blood, normally they are absent. In the human spleen nucleated red blood corpuscles are not to be found normally or in cases of severe anaemia, but exclusively in leukaemic diseases. U. Gabbi in his recently published work on the hæmolytic function of the spleen, also emphasises the difference between the various animal species. In guinea-pigs he found that the spleen acts largely as a scavenger of the red blood corpuscles; in rabbits very slightly. Consequently after removal of the spleen in guinea-pigs the number of red blood corpuscles rose 377,000 in the cubic millimetre, and the amount of hæmoglobin $8\cdot2\,^0/_0$. After splenectomy in rabbits the increase in these values is absent.

Shortly summarising our analysis of the facts before us, we must say that the importance of the spleen for the production of the white blood corpuscles can in no respect be considerable, and that if these cells really are produced by it, they must be free from granulations. The spleen therefore stands functionally in closer connection with the lymphatic gland system than with the bone-marrow. The spleen has not the least connection with ordinary leucocytosis[1].

## (β) The Lymphatic Glands.

As it is impossible experimentally to prevent the lymphatic glands as a whole from contributing to the formation of the blood, we are dependent almost entirely on clinical and anatomical researches for an elucidation of their function.

Since Virchow's definition of the lymphocyte it has been admitted that the lymphocytes of the blood, both the small and larger kinds, are identical with those of the lymphatic glands and the rest of the lymphatic system. This is proved by the complete agreement in general morphological character, in staining properties of the protoplasm and nucleus, and from the absence of granulation.

Abundant clinical experience testifies that the lymphocytes of the blood really do arise from the lymphatic system. Ehrlich had previously observed that when

---

[1] C. S. Engel has recently proposed to call acute leucocytosis "lienal leucocytosis," in analogy with the clinical idea of a lienal leukæmia. This terminology should only be used if the polynuclear cells did in fact arise from the spleen, an assumption which Engel himself does not once appear to make, since he expressly warns against drawing any conclusions from this name as to their origin. Since, however, the acute leucocytoses, as we shall shew in the next section, are exclusively to be referred to the bone-marrow, the term lienal leucocytosis seems to us quite mistaken, for it must logically lead to a conception of the origin of the leucocytes, exactly opposed to their actual relationships.

extensive portions of the lymphatic glandular system are put out of action by new growths and similar causes, the number of the lymphocytes may be considerably diminished. These observations have since that time been confirmed by various authors. For example, Reinbach describes several cases of malignant tumour, particularly sarcoma, in which the percentage of lymphocytes, which normally amounts to about 25 %, was very considerably lowered; in one case of lymphosarcoma of the neck they only made up 0·6 % of the total number. These conditions are quite easily and naturally explained by the exclusion of the lymphatic glands. It is difficult for the advocates of the view that the lymphocytes are the early stages of all white blood corpuscles to reconcile it with these facts. According to their scheme the low number of lymphocytes is to be explained in such cases by their unusually rapid transformation to the polynuclear elements—the old forms; or to appropriate the expression of Uskoff, by a too rapid ageing of the lymphocytes.

Further evidence for the origin of the lymphocytes of the blood from the lymphatic glands is to be obtained from those cases in which we find an increase of the lymphocytes in the blood. These "lymphocytoses" occur, in comparison with other leucocytoses, relatively seldom. Under certain conditions in which a hyperplasia of the lymphatic glandular apparatus makes its appearance, we often see at first an increase of the lymphocytes in the blood. Ehrlich and Karewski in some unpublished work have investigated together a large number of typical cases of lymphoma malignum, and were able constantly to observe a lymphocytosis, which in some cases was of high degree and bore almost a leukæmic character.

Relying on these facts Ehrlich and Wassermann (*Dermatolog. Zeitschr.* Vol. I., 1894) made the diagnosis *in vivo* of malignant lymphoma in a rare skin disease, chiefly from the absolute increase of the lymphocytes alone, although no swelling of the glands was palpable. The post-mortem shewed that the chief condition was a swelling of the retro-peritoneal lymph glands to lumps as large as a fist.

The lymphocytosis following extirpation of the spleen also belongs to this category, since a vicarious enlargement of the lymph glands is always to be observed in these cases.

On investigating the conditions under which in healthy individuals an increased number of lymphocytes enter the blood-stream, we have in the first place to notice the digestive canal, whose wall contains a thick layer of lymphatic tissue. According to the results of Rieder the proportion of the lymphocytes to polynuclears is practically normal in the leucocytosis of digestion, indeed the lymphocytes are rather in excess. The eosinophils on the other hand shew a marked relative reduction in this condition. The leucocytosis of digestion consequently differs essentially from the other kinds, in which the neutrophil elements are chiefly increased. The simultaneous increase of lymphocytes and polynuclears is doubtless brought about by a super-position of a raised income of lymphocytes, and an ordinary leucocytosis caused by the assimilated products of metabolism.

The influence of the digestive tract is still more evident in certain diseases, more particularly in intestinal diseases of infants. A considerable increase of the lymphocytes in the blood-stream is here to be observed. Thus Weiss found an important increase of the white blood corpuscles in simple catarrh of the stomach and intestines, which presented the main features of a lympho-cytosis.

Whooping-cough, according to the recent observations of Meunier, also belongs to the small number of diseases which are accompanied by a pronounced lymphæmia. In the convulsive period of this disease both the polynuclear cells and the lymphocytes are increased, the latter in preponderating amount. The former cells are increased to twice, the lymph cells to four times their normal amount. Doubtless in these cases also the lymphocytosis is due to the stimulation and swelling of the tracheo-bronchial glands.

An increase of the lymphocytes from chemical stimuli is exceedingly rare, though, as is well known, a large number of substances (bacterial products, proteins, nucleins, organic extracts, and so forth) can call forth a polynuclear leucocytosis. In quite isolated cases, an increase of the lymphocytes in the blood in consequence of the injection of tuberculin into tuberculous individuals has been seen. (E. Grawitz.) From the rarity of these cases it can scarcely be doubted that here a tuberculous disease of the glands also plays a part, so that the increased immigration of lymphocytes is brought about not by a chemical property of the tuberculin but by the extensive specific reaction of the diseased glands.

Only one single substance has so far been mentioned in the literature as capable in itself of producing a lym-phocytosis. Waldstein asserts that he has produced by injection of pilocarpine, a lymphæmia which undergoes a progressive increase with a rise in number of the injections.

The origin also of lymphocytosis is therefore sharply marked off from that of the ordinary leucocytosis, which consists in an increase of the neutrophil elements. Whilst the latter is admittedly the expression of chemiotactic action, and arises by action at a distance of soluble substances on the bone-marrow, lymphocytosis is due to a local stimulation of certain glandular areas. Thus in the leucocytosis of digestion, of intestinal diseases of children, we refer it to the excitation of the lymphatic apparatus of the intestine, in tuberculin lymphæmia we recognise mainly a reaction of the diseased lymph glands. Hence we conclude that a lymphocytosis appears when a raised lymph circulation occurs in a more or less extended area of lymphatic glands, and when, in consequence of the increased flow, more elements are mechanically washed out of the lymph glands. The pilocarpine lymphocytosis does not contradict this view, for pilocarpine causes extra-ordinary though transient variations in the distribution of water, whereby the inflow into the blood of fluid containing lymph cells is increased. We therefore re-gard lymphocytosis as the result of a mechanical process; whilst leucocytosis is the expression of an active chemiotactic reaction of the polynuclear elements.

This view finds its best support in the fact that the polynuclear leucocytes possess lively amœboid movement, which is completely wanting in the lymphocytes.

Corresponding to the absence of contractility in the lymphocytes it is also observed that in inflammatory processes in contradistinction to the polynuclear neutro- and oxyphils, the lymphocytes are not able to pass through the vessel wall. A very interesting experiment on this point was described by Neumann years ago. Neumann produced suppuration in a patient with lym-phatic leukæmia, in whom the blood contained only a very small number of polynuclear cells. Investigation of the pus shewed that it consisted exclusively of polynuclear cells, and that not a single lymphocyte had come into the exudation, although this kind of cell was present so abundantly in the blood.

Histological examination of all fresh inflammatory processes, in which mainly polynuclear elements are found, leads to accordant results. It is well known that small-celled infiltration occurs in the later stage of inflammation, apparently consisting of lymph cells; nevertheless this does not in the least prove that these lymphocytes have emigrated here from the blood vessels. This is not the place to enter into the very extensive controversy on this point. We are content to refer to the most recent very thorough paper of Ribbert. Ribbert regards these foci of small-celled infiltration as the analogues of the lymphatic nodules, and explains their origin by an increase in size of the foci of lymphatic tissue, normally present, though in a condition but little developed.

It consequently follows from clinical and morphological researches, as well as from the observations on inflammatory processes, that the lymphocytes are in no way connected with the polynuclear leucocytes. We shall reach the same result in another way in the following section.

## ($\gamma$)  **The Bone-marrow.**

The spleen and lymphatic glands were at first regarded as the sole places of formation of the blood corpuscles. The almost simultaneous researches of Neumann and Bizzozero first attracted general attention to the importance of the bone-marrow. These authors showed that the early stages of the red blood corpuscles are produced there; a discovery which was quickly and generally recognised, and which soon became pathologically useful through the observations of Cohnheim and others. In this connection the observation was of great value, that after severe loss of blood the fatty marrow of the larger hollow bones again changes to red marrow, as it is evidence of the increased demands on the regenerative function of the bone-marrow.

We are unaware of a second place of formation of the red blood corpuscles in man. In other mammalia however, as we have above mentioned (see page 99), the spleen may also take a small share in the production of erythrocytes. The type which the normal blood formation follows in adults, and the deviations therefrom shewn in pernicious anæmia, have been described in the chapter on the red blood corpuscles. Ehrlich's view that the blood formation in pernicious anæmia belongs to a different type, which is analogous to the embyronic, was also described there.

In this section we have therefore to deal chiefly with the white blood corpuscles and their connection with the bone-marrow. In man as in a large number of animals (for example the monkey, guinea-pig, rabbit, pigeon and so forth) the bone-marrow exhibits the peculiarity that the cells it produces bear a specific granulation, in sharp contrast to the lymphatic glandular system, which contains elements free from granules, in the whole animal series.

The granulated cells of the bone-marrow fall into two groups.

The first group of the cells with "special granules" is very important since it constitutes a characteristic for certain species of animals. According to the class of animal they shew different tinctorial and morphological properties. Man and monkey for example have neutrophil granulation; guinea-pig and rabbit the pseudo-eosinophil granulation described by Kurloff; in birds we find two specific granulations present side by side, which both are oxyphil, and of which one is imbedded in the protoplasm in crystalline form, the other in the form of granules.

The kinds of special granulations so far investigated have the common property, that they stain in acid and neutral dyes respectively; they shew a much smaller affinity for the basic dyes. The fact that they greatly exceed the other elements of the bone-marrow in all classes of animals, is evidence of the importance of these granules.

The second group of bone-marrow cells contains granules which we find in the whole vertebrate series from the frog to man, and which therefore are not characteristic for any one species of animal. They are, (1) the eosinophil cells, (2) the basophil mast cells.

The bone-marrow forms which are free from granules consist mostly of mononuclear cells of different type. They are not nearly so numerous, or so important as the granulated kind, more especially as the first and predominant group.

Amongst the granule-free forms the giant cells deserve special mention, for they are an almost constant constituent of the bone-marrow of the mammalian class. According to the recent researches of Pugliese the giant cells are considerably increased after extirpation of the spleen in the hedgehog; an organ of quite extraordinary size in this animal and doubtless therefore possessing important hæmatopoietic functions.

Pugliese asserts that in the hedgehog after splenectomy the nucleated giant cells pass into leucocytes by amitotic nuclear division. Unfortunately in his preliminary communication there are no notes of the granules of the bone-marrow cells.

On examining a stained dry preparation of the bone-marrow of the guinea-pig, rabbit, man, etc. it is seen that the characteristic finely granular cells are present in all stages of development, from the mononuclear through the transitional to the polynuclear (polymorphously nucleated) forms, which we meet with in the circulating blood. A glance at a preparation of this kind shews that the bone-marrow is clearly the factory where typical polynuclear cells are continuously formed from the granule-containing mononuclears.

Here also the same process of ripening can be seen in the polynuclear eosinophil leucocytes.

Ehrlich has been able by special differential staining to bring forward proof that the constitution of the granulation changes during the metamorphosis of the mononuclear to the polynuclear cells. In the young granules there is prominent a basophil portion that becomes less and less marked as the cell grows older. The pseudo-eosinophil granules of the mononuclear cells, of the guinea-pig for example, stain bluish-red in eosine-methylene blue after long fixing in superheated steam: in the transitional stages this admixture is gradually lost, and finally completely vanishes in the granules of the polynuclear leucocytes which stain pure red. Analogous observations may be made in the eosinophil cells of man and animals, and in the neutrophils of man. Hence it is even possible to decide whether an isolated granule belonged to an old or to a young cell.

It is still impossible to judge with certainty the rate at which the ripening of the mononuclear to the polynuclear cells proceeds, or further to decide if the ripening of the granules always runs parallel in point of time with that of the whole cell. On the grounds of our observations we would suppose that in general the two processes run their course side by side, but that in special cases the morphological ripening of the cell may proceed more rapidly than that of the granules. It is particularly easy to observe this point in eosinophil cells. Ehrlich had already mentioned in his first paper (1878) that side by side with the typical eosinophil granules isolated granules are often found which shew a deviation in tinctorial properties: for instance, they stain more of a black colour in eosine-aurantia-nigrosin; in eosine-methylene-blue, bluish-red to pure blue. Ehrlich had already described these as young elements in his first paper. The same differences are found more sharply marked in leukæmia even in the circulating blood, in the neutrophil as well as in the eosinophil group. Ehrlich has repeatedly found in leukæmic blood polynuclear eosinophil cells, whose granules must almost exclusively be regarded as young forms[1].

Ehrlich regarded these as typical examples of a relative acceleration of the morphological ripening of the cells, as compared with the development of the granules.

In normal blood we find only the ripe forms of the specific granulated cells of the bone-

[1] Many authors, e.g. Arnold, explain this double staining of the eosinophil cells by the presence of eosinophil and mast cell granulation side by side. That this is certainly not the case is shewn by the fact that the "basophil" granulation of the eosinophil cells does not in metachromatic staining shew the metachromasia characteristic for the mast cells.

marrow. The mononuclear and transitional forms of the neutrophil group, do not under normal circumstances pass over into the blood-stream.

Ehrlich regarded the mononuclear neutrophil granulated cells as characteristic for the bone-marrow, since they are found exclusively in the bone-marrow, never in the spleen or lymph glands, and for this reason named them "myelocytes," κατ᾽ ἔξοχην[1]. When myelocytes, no matter of what size, appear in considerable numbers in the blood of an adult, a leukæmia of myelogenic nature is nearly always present. (For the very rare exceptions to this rule, which it may be added can never be confused with leukæmia, see pages 77, 78.)

Exactly similar conditions hold good for the eosinophil cells, in as much as the singly nucleated forms, which one may call eosinophil myelocytes, occur, almost exclusively,

---

[1] A. Fränkel has recently reported histological investigations in which he could demonstrate in one case true myeloytes in inflamed lymph glands. He says (xv. *Congress f. innere Medecin*) : "For some time past I have had systematic examinations carried out by my assistant, Dr Japha, on the granulations of the leucocytes contained in these glands in a large number of infectious diseases, which are accompanied by acute swelling of the lymphatic glands, such as scarlet fever, diphtheria, typhoid. They were performed in the following way: dry coverslip preparations were made from the juice of the glands removed shortly after death, and were stained in the usual way by Ehrlich's triacid mixture. Amongst a large number of cases thus examined, it was possible in only one case of scarlet fever—but in this beyond all doubt— to demonstrate the presence of mononuclear cells with neutrophil granulation." The extreme rarity of this condition supports our opinion that the formation of neutrophil mononuclear elements cannot be regarded as a normal function of the lymphatic glands. Polynuclear neutrophil cells are nearly always naturally present in inflamed lymph glands, as a product of the inflammation which has immigrated there. Every pus preparation shews that the polynuclear neutrophil leucocytes can change in the tissues to mononuclear, and the isolated observations of Japha should be explained in this manner.

in leukæmic blood. These forms, which were first recognised by H. F. Müller, are however of less importance,
for in myelogenic leukæmia the chief part of the foreign
admixture of the blood is made up of Ehrlich's myelocytes.

Very important conclusions on the interesting question
of leucocytosis can be drawn from these observations.
Bearing in mind that polynuclear neutrophil cells are
developed and stored up only in the bone-marrow, that
in ordinary leucocytosis only the polynuclear forms are
increased in the blood-stream, it is evident that leucocytosis is purely a function of the bone-marrow, as
Ehrlich has always insisted with all distinctness. It is
only on this assumption that the frequently sudden
appearance of leucocytosis, as has so often been observed
in morbid and experimental conditions, can be satisfactorily explained. In these cases the space of time,
amounting often only to minutes, is far too short for a
new formation of leucocytes to be conceivable; there
must be places in which these cells are already completely
formed, and able thence to emigrate on any suitable
stimulus. This place is single, and is the bone-marrow
alone. Here all mononuclear forms gradually ripen to
the polynuclear contractile cells, which obey each chemiotactic stimulus by emigration, and which thus bring about
sudden leucocytosis.

The bone-marrow thus fulfils, amongst others, the
extremely important function of a protective organ, by
which definite injurious influences which affect the organism may be quickly and energetically combated.
Just as in a fire-station ample means of assistance is
continuously in readiness immediately to answer an alarm
from any quarter.

We wish to insist once more, that the large mononuclear leucocytes and the transitional forms of the
normal blood are not concerned in the increase in ordinary
leucocytosis; in leucocytosis of high degree their relative
number may indeed be lowered, in consequence of the
exclusive increase of the polynuclear cells. It appears
then that these elements do not react to chemiotactic
stimuli, and that possibly they reach the blood by entirely different ways than the polynuclears do.

We believe that these non-granulated mononuclear cells of man
are to be regarded as analogous to those of the guinea-pig described
by Kurloff (see page 86). The mononuclear cells of man however
are finally transformed into the neutrophil granulated cells, whilst
the cells of Kurloff remain free from granules in the course of their
metamorphosis. In acute leucocytosis in the guinea-pig only the
pseudo-eosinophil polynuclear cells are increased, which wander as
such out of the bone-marrow, but not the polynucleated non-
granulated forms, which but slowly grow to maturity in the blood.
Thus the peculiarities of guinea-pig's blood, in which two kinds of
polynuclear cells are recognisable, throw light upon the corresponding
conditions in human blood. The distinction in the latter is more
difficult, since it is not evident in this case that the fully formed
polynuclear neutrophil leucocytes have a twofold origin : for the
majority wander fully formed from the bone-marrow into the
blood, and only a considerably smaller number grow to maturity
within the blood-stream from the mononuclear and transitional
forms.

No definite statement can as yet be made as to the
places of formation of the non-granulated large mononuclear leucocytes.

Kurloff has demonstrated, that in the guinea-pig these
cells are present both in the bone-marrow and in the
spleen, but that after extirpation of the spleen the
absolute number does not change. The bone-marrow

then in the guinea-pig can also preserve the balance of the large mononuclear, non-granular cells in the blood.

The numbers we found in our blood investigations in man after splenectomy were also normal. We may then doubtless assume that the large mononuclear granuleless cells of human blood also arise for the most part from the bone-marrow. In this tissue they are to be picked out in the medley of the different kinds of cells only with the utmost difficulty, owing to their small number and their but little characteristic properties. Consequently an exact investigation of their origin could probably only be successful if it were possible experimentally to produce a disease in which these forms in particular underwent important increase. This advance is not quite hopeless, since in man at least an absolute increase of the large mononuclear cells is observed in the post-febrile stage of measles.

On the grounds merely of microscopical investigations we conclude that the bone-marrow is by far the most important of the blood-forming organs, for its function is the exclusive production of red blood discs as well as of the chief group of the white corpuscles, the polynuclear neutrophil.

The physiological, experimental investigation of the functions of the bone-marrow offers insurmountable difficulties. An exclusion of the whole bone-marrow or of larger portions only is an impossible operation. Nor can we ascribe any value to the researches which endeavour to obtain a result by comparative enumerations of the arterial and venous blood of a bone-marrow area. J. P. Roietzky working under Uskoff's direction has recently made counts of this kind in the dog, from the nutrient artery of the tibia and the corresponding vein.

He found that the number of white corpuscles of the vein is slightly greater, that on the other hand the absolute number of "young corpuscles" (Uskoff), *i.e.* of the lymphocytes, has been considerably diminished, whilst the number of "ripe" corpuscles, which for the most part correspond to our polynuclear, is considerably increased. He gives the following table:

| Total number | Young corpuscles | Ripe corpuscles | Old corpuscles |
|---|---|---|---|
| Arterial blood 15000 | 1950 (13 %) | 840 (5·6 %) | 12210 (81 %) |
| Venous    ,,    16400 | 656 (4·0 %) | 2788 (17·0 %) | 12956 (79·0 %) |

The argument based on figures such as these assumes that the function of the bone-marrow is continuous; an assumption which Uskoff indeed seems to make.

But if the bone-marrow is constantly absorbing the lymphocytes to such an extent, it is quite incomprehensible how the normal condition of the blood can be preserved, bearing in mind the extent of the bone-marrow and the rate of the circulation. All evidence indeed tends to shew that on the contrary the bone-marrow performs its functions discontinuously, inasmuch as elements continually grow to maturity in the bone-marrow, as we have above explained, but they only emigrate at certain times as the result of chemical stimuli. It is obvious *a priori* from this consideration how inconclusive must be the results of experiments such as these of Roietzky[1].

---

[1] Moreover the investigations of Roietzky are quite without foundation, inasmuch as the tibia of the dog, upon which this author performed his experiments, contains in all races of dogs—according to the information very kindly given us by Prof. Schütz—no red marrow, but fatty marrow only, which as is well known is incapable of the smallest hæmatopoietic function.

Far more important for the elucidation of the function of the bone-marrow are clinical observations on cases in which considerable portions of the bone-marrow are replaced by tissue of another kind.  We may best divide the observations on this point into two groups: 1. malignant tumours of the bone-marrow, 2. the so-called acute leukæmia.

There are unfortunately very few available observations as yet upon the first group.  Still rarer are the cases in which as is necessary the whole bone-marrow has been subjected to an exhaustive examination, which alone affords adequate evidence of the extent of the defect.

Amongst the changes of the bone-marrow arising from tumours one may distinguish two groups, according to the nature of the condition of the blood.  The first type is exemplified by a case of Nothnagel published in his work on lymphadenia ossium.  Here during life the blood shewed, in the main, the features of a simple severe anæmia; but in addition isolated normoblasts, small marrow cells, and moderate leucocytosis.  The autopsy, at which the whole skeletal system was subjected systematically to an exact examination, shewed a complete atrophy of the bone-marrow, and replacement of the same by the tumour masses.  In this case then the condition of the blood *in vivo* is satisfactorily explained by the absence of function of bone-marrow.  Nothnagel conjectured that the formation of the scanty nucleated red blood corpuscles occurred vicariously in the spleen, that of the leucocytes in the lymph glands.

In the second series to which the cases of Israel and Leyden, as well as the recently published one of J. Epstein from Neusser's wards, belong, the blood shews, besides the usual anæmic changes, other anomalies which are peculiar

partly to pernicious anæmia, partly to myelogenic leukæmia. In Epstein's case of metastatic carcinoma of the
bone-marrow, there was found a considerable anæmia,
with numerous nucleated red blood corpuscles both of
the normo- and megalo-blastic type; their nuclei presented the strangest shapes, due not merely to typical
nuclear division, but also to nuclear degeneration. The
white blood corpuscles were much increased, their
proportion to the red was $\frac{1}{25}$ to $\frac{1}{40}$; the increase concerned in the main the large mononuclear forms, which
bore for the most part neutrophil granulation, and were
therefore to be called myelocytes. In all the specimens,
only two eosinophil cells were found[1].

The explanation of a blood picture of this kind, apart
from the purely anæmic changes, is by no means easy, as
Epstein rightly observes. The appearance of myelocytes
is most readily explained by a direct stimulation of the
remaining bone-marrow by the surrounding masses of
tumour. In this, the mechanical factor is less concerned
than the chemical metabolic products of the tumour
masses; which at first act on the adjacent tissue in
specially strong concentration, and also in a negatively
chemiotactic manner on the wandering cells. This view
receives support from the careful work of Reinbach on
the behaviour of the leucocytes in malignant tumours.
Out of 40 cases examined, in only one, of lymphosarcoma
complicated with tuberculosis, were myelocytes found in
the blood, amounting to about 0·5—1·0 % of the white
blood corpuscles. The autopsy shewed isolated yellowish
white foci of growth in the bone-marrow, reaching the

---

[1] We draw particular attention to the small number of eosinophil
cells, since according to Ehrlich's postulates this absence of eosinophil
cells is incompatible with the diagnosis of a leukæmia.

size of a sixpenny piece. Bearing in mind that in none of the other 39 cases were myelocytes demonstrated, one does not hesitate to explain their presence in the blood in this single case by the metastases in the bone-marrow. The small extent of the latter is likewise the cause of the small percentage of the myelocytes.

In explaining the presence of the megaloblasts in the blood of Epstein's patient we must keep before us what we have said elsewhere on this kind of cell. They are not present in the normal bone-marrow; they arise on the contrary, according to our view, when a specific morbid agent acts upon the bone-marrow, as we must assume is the case in the pernicious forms of anæmia. In the cases of anæmia from tumours, in which we find megaloblasts in large numbers in the blood, we must likewise assume that chemical stimuli proceed from the tumours, leading to the formation of megaloblasts in the bone-marrow.

The presence of megaloblasts in the bone-marrow does not itself cause their appearance in the blood, for in pernicious anæmia the bone-marrow may be filled with megaloblasts, and yet only very scanty examples are to be found in the blood. Whether the emigration of the megaloblasts from the bone-marrow into the blood-stream is in general to be referred to chemical stimuli, as it is in the particular case of Epstein's, or to mechanical causes, cannot at present be decided.

The bone-marrow may be replaced by typical lymphatic tissue, as well as by the substance of malignant tumours. The former occurs constantly in lymphatic leukæmia according to the well-known results of Neumann, which have since been generally confirmed. In these cases extensive tracts of bone-marrow are replaced not by masses of malignant growth but by an indifferent tissue, so to speak, a tissue which is unable to exercise the above-described stimulating influence upon the remaining bone-marrow. It is owing to this circumstance that we are able to observe in the cases of lymphatic degeneration of the bone-marrow the phenomena due to its exclusion, in their most uncomplicated form[1].

The most convincing results are obtained from cases of acute (lymphatic) leukæmia, the pretty frequent occurrence of which was first noticed by Epstein, and which has lately been very thoroughly studied by A. Fränkel, For the purpose in question, acute leukæmia is specially suited, since the abnormal growth of the lymphatic tissue takes place very rapidly, and for this reason brings about a quick and uncomplicated exclusion of the bone-marrow tissue; as it were, experimentally. Under its influence the neutrophil elements of the bone-marrow vanish rapidly, and in many cases so completely that it needs some trouble to find a single myelocyte, as for example in a case of Ehrlich's. The polynuclear leucocytes are produced in the bone-marrow, consequently where the bone-marrow is destroyed, as in this case, it is clear that their numbers must be absolutely very much diminished in the blood.

Dock has also arrived at similar results, as we see from a preliminary report; and he similarly explains the absence of neutrophil cells in lymphatic leukæmia by the replacement of the myeloid by lymphatic tissue.

[1] In contrast to this lymphatic metamorphosis of the bone-marrow, in myelogenous leukæmia a myeloid transformation of the other blood-forming organs, especially of the lymph glands is found; a transformation sufficiently characterised as myeloid by the presence of myelocytes, eosinophils, and nucleated red blood corpuscles.

Thus lymphatic leukæmia affords a striking proof that the lymphocytes are cells of a peculiar kind, and which are quite independent of the polynuclear cells. It is therefore exceedingly surprising that Fränkel, after accurately examining and analysing eight cases of acute lymphatic leukæmia, believes he has found in them imperative reasons for the assumption that the lymphocytes are transformed to polynuclear cells. This can only be explained by the confusion which Uskoff's doctrine of "young cells" has brought about.

We define lymphocytosis as an increase of the lymphocytes of the blood; Fränkel like Uskoff regards it as the emigration of the young forms of the white blood corpuscles into the blood. He concludes logically from the diminution of the polynuclear cells in this form of disease "that the conditions of the transformation of the young forms have undergone a disturbance." But if one assumes that the lymphocytes are young forms, and the polynuclears their older stages, it is much nearer to the facts to speak, not of a disturbance in lymphatic leukæmia, but of an absolute hinderance to the ripening process. It is easy to conceive any particular stimulus or injury bringing about an acceleration of the normal process, that is, a premature old age, but it is equally difficult to represent clearly to oneself conditions which retard or completely prevent the normal ageing of the elements. The discovery of such conditions would be really epoch-making, both for general biology, and for therapeutics. The only escape from this dilemma would be the assumption of a very premature death of the lymphocytes, for which however not the smallest evidence is to be found, even in Fränkel's monograph. Frankel distinguishes the acute from the chronic forms of leukæmia by the fact, "that in the former the newly formed elements emigrate from their places of formation into the blood-stream with extraordinary rapidity. Hence there is not time for further local metamorphosis. In chronic leukæmia the emigration takes place very probably much more slowly." This distinction is contradicted by the facts; for there are chronic forms of lymphatic leukaemia whose microscopic picture is identical with that of acute leukaemia. And hence the starting-point of all Fränkel's deductions is rendered insecure.

## III. ON THE DEMONSTRATION OF THE CELL-
## GRANULES, AND THEIR SIGNIFICANCE.

DURING the last ten years a large amount of valuable work has been done on the cell-granules from histological, biological and clinical sides. This has particularly assisted hæmatology, where a number of problems remain whose solution is only possible by the aid of a knowledge of the granules. We must therefore consider the history, methods, and results of this work.

Ehrlich was undoubtedly the first to insist on the importance of the cell-granules, and to obtain practical results in this direction. We are obliged to mention this, since Altmann has, in spite of express corrections, repeatedly asserted the contrary. In 1891[1] Ehrlich refuted Altmann's claim to priority, nevertheless, Altmann in the 2nd edition of his *Elementary Organisms* (1894) stated that before him no one had recognised the specific importance of the granules, though some authors had viewed them as "rare and isolated phenomena."

We may quote a passage published by Ehrlich in 1878[2],

[1] *Farbenanalytische Untersuchungen* XII: *zur Geschichte der Granula*, p. 134.

[2] *loc. cit.* pp. 5, 6.

that is, ten years before Altmann's papers. "Since the beginning of histology the word 'granular' has been used to describe the character of cellular forms. This term is not a very happy one, since many circumstances produce a granular appearance of the protoplasm. Modern work has shewn that many cells, formerly described as granular, owe this appearance to a reticular protoplasmic framework. And we have no more right to call cells granular in which proteid precipitates occur, either spontaneously as in coagulation, or from reagents (alcohol). The name should be kept exclusively for cells in which during life substances, chemically distinct from normal proteid, are embedded in a granular form. We can readily distinguish but few of these substances, such as fat and pigment; most of them we can at present characterise but imperfectly, or not at all."

"Earlier observations, especially on the mast cells, led me to expect that these granulations, though they had long been inaccessible to chemical analysis, could be distinguished by their behaviour with certain stains. I found, in fact, granules of this kind, characterised by their affinity for certain dyes, and which could thereby be easily followed through the animal series and in various organs. I further found that certain granules only occurred in particular cells, for which they were characteristic, as pigment is for pigment cells, and glycogen for cartilage cells (Neumann) and so forth. We can diagnose the variously shaped mast cells only by the staining of their granules in dahlia solution, that is by a microchemical test. And in the same way we can separate tinctorially other granulated cells, morphologically indistinguishable, into definite sub-groups. And for this reason, I propose to call these granulations specific."

"The investigations were performed after Koch's method in the following manner. The fluid (blood) or the parenchyma of the organs (bone-marrow, spleen, etc.) was spread on coverslips in as thin a layer as possible, dried at room temperature, and after a convenient length of time stained. I had chosen this apparently coarse method for the special reason that for the histological recognition of new, possibly definite chemical combinations, corresponding to the granulations, all substances must be avoided that might act as solvents, e.g. water or alcohol, or as oxydising agents, such as osmic acid. In this instance only such procedures may be employed as will leave the simple drying of each single chemical substance as much as possible unchanged."

A more detailed study of the process of staining, and of the relation between chemical constitution and staining power, enabled a further advance to be made. And the first result in this previously unworked direction, was the sharp distinction between acid, basic, and neutral dyes, and between the corresponding, oxy-, baso-, and neutrophil granulations. The triacid solution was only found after trial of many hundred combinations; and up to the present day this stain in its original form or in slight modifications has played a prominent part in various provinces of histology.

The classification of the cell-granules of the blood according to their various chemical affinities which was drawn up by this method is accepted to-day as the most valuable, and the only practical means of grouping the leucocytes. From the first Ehrlich has insisted, that different kinds of cells possess different granules, distinguished not only by their tinctorial properties, but also by their various reactions to solvents.

It is in this connection indeed, that Altmann's method, consisting of a complicated hardening process, and the use of a single, always similar stain, constitutes a retrograde step, in as much as it tends to obscure the principle of the specificity of each kind of granulation.

A further disadvantage of Altmann's hardening method lies in the circumstance, that the cell proteids are precipitated by it in a spherical form, and stain in the subsequent treatment. Hence it is extremely difficult to distinguish what is preformed, and what is artefact. Since A. Fischer's publication, where the formation of granule-like precipitates under the influence of various reagents is experimentally demonstrated, grave doubts as to the reality of Altmann's forms have been raised from various quarters. Ehrlich's dry process, on the contrary, is entirely free from error. Granules cannot be artificially produced, by desiccation, and the stained appearances correspond precisely to what is seen in fresh living blood. The greatest value of the dry method is that the chemical nature of the single granules remains unchanged, so that attempts at differentiation are made on a nearly unaltered object[1].

Another means of studying the nature of the granules depends on the principle of vital staining. The " vital methylene blue staining " (Ehrlich) that has since become so important, especially in neurology, led to the first attempts at staining the granules in living animals. One of the first publications on this subject is that of O. Schultze, who placed the larvæ of frogs in dilute methylene blue solution, and after a short period found

[1] Altmann's freezing process would be similar to the advance always insisted on by Ehrlich. It offers such great technical difficulties, however, that it has up to now been little used.

the granules of the stomach, the red blood corpuscles and other cells stained blue. This method, however, cannot pass as entirely free from error, as Ehrlich frequently found that when the experiment lasts some time the methylene blue often forms granular precipitates that may be confused with the granules. Teichmann directs a detailed analysis to this point, and regards most of the granules described by Schultze as artificial products.

Neutral red is highly suitable for the study of vital granule-staining, a dye recommended by Ehrlich, and employed successfully since that time by Przesmycki, Prowazek, S. Mayer, Solger, Friedmann, Pappenheim and others. This dye was prepared by O. N. Witt from nitrosodimethylamin and metatoluylendiamin, and is the hydrochloric acid salt of a base which is soluble in pure water, yielding a fuchsin red colour, but which in weak alkaline solution—the alkalinity of mineral water suffices— is a yellow-orange hue.

Now neutral red is characterised by a really maximal affinity for the majority of the granules. Ehrlich was able by the aid of this dye to demonstrate granules, even in some vegetable cells. Moreover the method of using it is the simplest conceivable, as subcutaneous or intravenous injection, or even feeding, in the higher animals stains the granules; with frog's larvæ and invertebrates, to allow them to swim in a dilute solution of the dye is often sufficient. The staining also succeeds in "surviving" organs, and is best effected by allowing small pieces to float in physiological salt solution, to which a trace of neutral red is added, under plentiful access of air. When the object is macroscopically red it is ready for examination.

The finest results are naturally given by organs that are easily teased out, *e.g.* flies' eggs, or the Malpighian canals of insects. The staining solution is to be chosen so that the act of staining does not last too long, but on the other hand too high a concentration must not be used. About $\frac{1}{50000}$ to $\frac{1}{100000}$ is recommended, so that the protoplasm and nucleus remain quite uncoloured. Artificial products with this method cannot entirely be excluded, and, *e.g.* in plant-cells containing tannin, are to be explained by the production and precipitation of the salt of tannic acid. However it is not difficult for the experienced to recognise artificial products as such in individual cases. The kind of granulation, the typical distribution, a comparison with neighbouring cells, the combination of various methods, the comparison of the same object under vital and "survival" staining, facilitate judgment and obviate mistakes of this kind.

The majority of the granules of vertebrates are stained orange-red by neutral red, corresponding with the weakly alkaline reaction of these forms. Granules staining in pure fuchsin colour and which hence possess a weak acid reaction are much more rarely found.

Combination staining may be recommended as a valuable aid to the neutral red method. Ehrlich has used a double stain with neutral red and methylene blue. Frog's larvæ were allowed to remain in a solution of neutral red, to which a trace of methylene blue had been added. He then found red granulations almost exclusively, only the granules of the smooth musculature of the stomach were stained intensely blue. With the aid of a threefold combination Ehrlich obtained a still further differentiation of the living cell-granules. There is no doubt whatever that a thorough study of this neutral red method would lead to important conclusions as to the nature and function of the granules, and lead us to the most real problems of cell life. With our present information even we can get definite conceptions founded upon facts, as to the biological importance of the cell-granules.

---

In his first publication Ehrlich described the granules as products of the metabolism of the cells, deposited within the protoplasm in a solid form, in part to serve as reserve material, in part to be cast off from the cell. On the ground of observations on the liver cells, described in detail in a paper of Frerichs (1883, page 43), Ehrlich gave up this position, though only temporarily. Ehrlich shewed that the liver cells of a rabbit's liver, rich in glycogen, appear in dry preparations as bulky polygonous elements, of a uniform homogeneous brown colour, surrounded by a thin, well-defined yellow membrane. In cells that were not too rich in glycogen, small roundish bodies, clearly of a protoplasmic nature, of a pure yellow, can be seen embedded in the homogeneous cells that are coloured brown with glycogen. "The hyaline cellular ground substance, carrying the glycogen, could not under any circumstances be stained, but the cell-granules above mentioned stained easily with all kinds of dyes. It was further possible to shew by staining that the membrane was chemically different from the granules, since with eosin-aurantia-indulin-glycerine, the membrane stained black, but the granules orange-red."

To these observations Ehrlich added the following conclusion, "that the cells of the liver after food really possess a thin protoplasmic membrane, and a homogeneous glycogen-bearing substance, in which the nucleus and round granules (? functionally active) of protoplasm are embedded.

"On comparing these results with those of more recent investigation of the cells, it is easy to determine the location of the glycogen very accurately. Kupffer has shewn, first for the liver cells—and this is now recognised as generally valid—that their contents do not represent a microscopically single substance. In the 'survival' preparation he found, in addition to the nucleus, two clearly distinct substances: a hyaline ground substance in preponderating amount, and a more scanty, finely granular, fibrillary substance embedded in it. Kupffer calls the first paraplasm, the latter protoplasm. On warming the preparation to about 22° C. manifest though feeble movements appeared in the network. It can hardly be doubted, that of these two substances the granular reticulated one—the protoplasm—is the more important; and it should not be erroneous to suppose that the granulations of the network form the centre of the particular (specific) cell function. In any case, it is desirable to give a special name, such as microsomes (Hanstein) to these forms, which in the liver cells are recognisable as distinct, round or oval granules, colouring yellow with iodine, and easily and deeply staining in other ways."

It was necessary to quote in full from this older paper, to shew that Ehrlich regarded the granules as the special carriers of the cell function so long ago as 1883, a view that Altmann advocated many years later, under the name "theory of bioblasts." Altmann's ever repeated assertion that no one before him had allotted so high an importance to the granules is consequently in disagreement with the facts we have above made sufficiently clear.

The importance Altmann ultimately gave to the granules, which he also calls by the name "Ozonophores" is shewn by his own words (*Elementary Organisms*, 1st edit., p. 39):

"Our conception of the ozonophores may therefore replace that of the living protoplasm, at least so far as vegetative function is concerned; and may serve us as an explanation of complicated organic processes. Once again, shortly summarising the properties of the ozonophores; as oxygen carriers they can perform reduction and oxydation, and can thus effect the decompositions and syntheses of the body, without losing their own individuality."

In the meantime Ehrlich had made various observations which could not be completely brought into line with his own earlier hypothesis or the far-reaching conclusions of Altmann. Studies in particular on the oxygen requirements of the organism, shewed that the "ozonophores" could certainly not be an important part of the cell. In addition it was found that normally cells occur in which no granules can be recognised by ordinary methods. Finally a pathological observation made untenable the view that the granules are the bearers of the cell function. In a case of pernicious anæmia (cp. *Farbenanalytische untersuchungen*) Ehrlich found the polynuclear cells of the blood and bone-marrow and their early forms free from all neutrophil granulation. On the grounds of this observation Ehrlich returned to his original assumption that the granules are secretory products of the cells, and defined his standpoint at that time as follows:

"Did the neutrophil granulations really represent the bodies which supply these cells with oxygen, as Altmann supposes, a condition such as we have here brought

forward would be impossible, since with the disappearance of the granules death of the cells must follow.  But
from the point of view of the secretion theory the
condition described is easily explainable.  Just as under
certain conditions fat-cells may completely lose their
contents without dying, so the bone-marrow cell, if the
blood fails to yield to it the necessary substances, may
occasionally be unable to produce more neutrophil granules.
And thus it becomes non-granular."

The view, that the granules are special metabolic
products of the specific cellular activity, is strongly
supported by the great chemical differences between
them.  Ehrlich made these peculiarities clear for the
blood-cells, and found that their granulations differ from
one another, not only in their colour reactions, but also
in their shape and solubility; so that they must be
sharply distinguished.

Whilst for instance the majority of the granules are
more or less rounded forms, in some classes of animals,
e.g. in birds, the analogues of the granules of mammalian
blood are characterised by a decided crystalline form, and
a strong oxyphilia.  The substance of the mast cell granulations is also crystalline in some species of animals.

The size of the individual granules is constant in any
animal species for every kind of granule—excepting only
the mast cells.  The eosinophil granulation reaches its
greatest size in the horse, where really gigantic examples
are found.

The presence of granulated colourless blood-cells has
been demonstrated in the most various classes of animals,
and even in the blood of many invertebrates, particularly,
as Knoll has shewn, in the Lamellibranchiates, Polychætes,
Pedates, Tunicates and Cephalopods.  Concerning verte-

brates, especially the higher classes, accurate and ample researches are to hand. In birds we recognise two oxyphil granulations, of which one is embedded in the cells in the crystalline, the other in the usual granular form. Amongst the vertebrates most investigated classes possess granulated polynuclear cells. To this circumstance Hirschfeld has recently devoted a thorough paper containing many details worthy of note. In the majority of the animals observed, he found too that the polynuclear cells contained neutrophil granules; in only one animal, the white mouse, did he find them, or granulations analogous to them, completely wanting.

According to the investigations carried out some years back in Ehrlich's laboratory by Dr Franz Müller, these results of Hirschfeld's must be described as inaccurate. After many vain endeavours, Dr Müller was able to find a method by which numerous though very minute granules could be found in the polynuclear cells of the mouse. The case shews that it is not permissible to assume the absence of granules, when the ordinary staining methods are not at once successful. There is no universal method for the staining of granules, any more than for the staining of various kinds of bacteria. Indeed all granules, that are easily soluble, vanish when the triacid method is used, and so a homogeneous cell protoplasm is simulated.

But naturally, the occurrence of non-granulated polynuclear cells in certain classes of animals is not to be denied from these considerations. Hirschfeld asserts that such cells occur side by side with granulated cells, for instance in the dog; and draws from them far-reaching conclusions as to the meaning of the granules. From Kurloff's work (see p. 85) we must insist, on the contrary,

that there is no evidence that the non-granulated polynuclears are identical with the granulated cells. Kurloff
has shewn, at least for guinea-pig's blood, that these two
heterogeneous elements are to be sharply separated one
from the other, and that they have an entirely different
origin.

Specially important for a theory of the nature of the
granules is the circumstance, that generally speaking in
all species of animals they are present in those cells
of the blood only which are adapted to and capable
of emigration. That a certain nutritive function is to
be ascribed to the emigration of the granulated cells is
a very obvious supposition, scarcely to be denied; and
naturally cells with a plentiful store of reserve material
are eminently suited for this purpose. The lymphocytes
on the contrary, incapable of emigration, are almost
totally devoid of specific granulations.

A further indication that the granulations really
are connected with a specific cell activity lies in
the fact, that one cell bears but one specific granulation. The contrary assertions that neutrophil and
eosinophil, or eosinophil and mast cell granulations occur
in the same cell Ehrlich regards as unfounded, from
extensive researches specially directed to this point. Nor
has Ehrlich seen a pseudoeosinophil cell of the rabbit
change to a true eosinophil[1]. That such a transition

---

[1] The cause of these misunderstandings is the tinctorially different
stages of development of the granules, as we have fully explained above.
How little adequate tinctorial differences by themselves are to settle the
chemical identity of a granulation, is at once evident on consideration of
the granules of other organs. No one surely would assert, that a
liver, muscle, or brain cell could occasionally secrete trypsin, simply
because the granules of the pancreas stain similarly and analogously to
those of the cells mentioned. We would here expressly insist that we

does not occur is most distinctly shewn by the fact that the various granulations behave entirely differently towards solvents. With the aid of acids, for example, the pseudoeosinophil granules can be completely extracted from the cells, whilst the eosinophil granules remain whole under this process, and can now be stained by themselves.

The clearest proof that the neutrophil, eosinophil, and mast cells are entirely separated from one another by the fundamental diversity of their protoplasm, of which the granulation is but a specially striking expression, is afforded by the study of the various forms of leucocytosis. As will be shewn in detail in the following chapter, neutrophil and eosinophil leucocytes behave quite differently in their susceptibility to chemiotactic stimulation. Substances strongly positively or negatively chemiotactic for one cell group are as a rule indifferent for the other; frequently indeed there is an exactly opposed relationship, inasmuch as substances which attract the one kind repel the other. Still greater is the difference between the mast cells and the other two cell groups; for so far as present investigations go, they are quite uninfluenced by substances chemiotactic for the neutrophil or eosinophil cells.

As specific cellular secretions, various kinds of granules must also be sharply marked off from each other by their chemical properties. The granules of the blood corpuscles seem to be of very simple chemical constitution.

only assume a distinct character for each kind of granulation, in the strict sense of the term for the cells of the blood, since they possess a relatively simple function. In very complex glandular cells, however, with various simultaneous functions, several kinds of granules may be contained.

We have special grounds for the assumption that the crystalline granulations are for the most part composed of a single chemical compound, not necessarily highly complex even, but which seems to be a relatively simple body such as guanin, fat, melanin, etc. Doubtless other granulations have a more complicated constitution, and very often are a mixture of various chemical substances. The most complicated granules of the blood are the eosinophil, which are, as has elsewhere already been mentioned, of a more complex histological structure. For a peripheral layer is plainly distinguishable from the central part of the granule. It should be mentioned that according to Barker the eosinophil granulations appear to contain iron.

The key-stone of the hypothesis of the secretory nature of the granules is the direct observation of a secretory process in the cells bearing the granules. Naturally these researches offer extraordinary difficulties since only the coincidence of a number of lucky circumstances would allow the passage of dissolved granule substance into the neighbourhood to be followed. Kanthack and Hardy have succeeded in demonstrating the secretory nature of the eosinophil granules of the frog. When, for example, anthrax bacilli are introduced into the dorsal lymph sac of the frog they exert a positive chemiotaxis on the eosinophil cells. The latter come in contact with the bacilli, and remain for some time attached to them. During this period Kanthack and Hardy observed a discharge of granules from these cells, which now possess a protoplasm relatively homogeneous. Afterwards these cells move away from the bacilli, and are succeeded by the polynuclear neutrophil cells, as will be mentioned later. These authors were further able to observe gradual accumulation of granules in eosinophil cells in lymph kept under microscopic observation as a hanging drop, and thus demonstrated that they undergo the two stages characteristic of secretion, (1) appearance of granules within the cells, (2) discharge of these granules externally.

The mast cells too seem suited for this purpose since their specific substance is strongly characterised by its peculiar metachromatic staining, and is further especially readily recognisable, since by its great affinity for basic dyes it remains plainly stained, even in preparations that are almost quite decolorised. In fact appearances of the mast cells are not infrequently found, which must be referred to excretory processes of this kind.

In the first place it is occasionally seen that the mast cell granulation is dissolved within the cell, and diffuses in solution into the nucleus. In place of the well-known picture of the mast cell (see page 76) of a colourless nucleus, surrounded by a deeply stained metachromatic granulation, a nucleus is present intensely and homogeneously stained in the tint of the mast cell granulation, surrounded by a protoplasm shewing but traces of granules.

Still more convincing is the presence of a peculiar halo of the mast cells, described by various authors. Ehrlich first shortly mentioned this halo in his book on the oxygen requirements of the organism. A few years ago, Unna, whose notice Ehrlich's remark had no doubt escaped, described an analogous condition as follows: "in some nodules the mast cells appeared in part twice as large as usual, especially with the new mast cell stain (polychrome methylene blue, glycerine ether mixture). This was caused by the staining of a large round halo, in the centre of which lay the peculiar long-known mast cell, consisting of blue nucleus, and an areola of deep red granules. Higher magnification shewed that the halo was not granular, but very finely reticular; although it exhibited exactly the same red colour as the granules. It was consequently a spongioplasm peculiar to these mast cells."

The appearance of the mast cells described by Unna may also be artificially produced, by allowing a preparation that is stained with the oxygen containing analogue of thionin, oxamine, to remain for some time in lævulose syrup or watery glycerine. Evidently part of the dyed mast cell substance is dissolved and retained in the immediate neighbourhood. But as Unna possesses great experience of the mast cells and is a complete master of the methods of their demonstration, one must suppose that the halos described by him were preformed, and did not arise during the preparation of the specimen.

It must hence be concluded that an analogous process may go on during life, that these halos are the expression of a vital secretion of the substance of the mast cells externally[1].

A condition that Prus has brought forward in the so-called purpura of the horse, is also to be interpreted as a secretory process of the mast cells. He describes young mast cells from the hæmorrhagic foci of the wall of the gut, on the margins of which bodies of

[1] From a paper of Calleja we learn that Ramon y Cajal recognised the halos of the mast cells, and interpreted them in the manner we have above. Calleja also describes these halos and the method of demonstrating them in detail (thionin staining, and mounting the sections in glycerine). We must mention, however, that we do not consider this method suitable for the recognition of preformed halos, for the reasons above mentioned.

various sizes appeared, and which differ essentially from
the mast cells themselves by their staining. Nevertheless
from their whole configuration and position it is evident
that these bodies have arisen in the mast cells themselves; and Prus comes to the conclusion "that the
degenerating young mast cells secrete a fluid or
semi-fluid substance, which as a rule sets on the
surface of the cells, but also, more rarely, in their
interior."

Evidence that the substance of the granules is given
off externally may sometimes be seen in the polynuclear
neutrophil or their analogues. Thus in rabbit's blood
in which he had experimentally produced leucocytosis,
Hankin found a distinct progressive decrease of the
pseudoeosinophil granules on allowing the samples of
blood to remain some time in the thermostat. Further
in suppurating foci in man, especially when suppuration
has lasted long, or the pus has remained for some time in
the place in question (Janowski) a rarefaction almost to
complete disappearance of the polynuclear neutrophil
granules occurs, and is to be explained by a giving up
of the granulations to the exterior.

These facts and considerations, on the whole, lead then
to the conclusion, that in general the granules of the
wandering cells are destined for excretion. This
elimination of the granules is probably one of
the most important functions of the polynuclear
leucocytes.

## IV. LEUCOCYTOSIS.

THE problem of leucocytosis is one of the most keenly debated questions of modern medicine. An exhaustive account of the various works devoted to it, of the methods and results, could fill by itself a whole volume, and would widely exceed the limits of an account of the histology of the blood. We can only deal fully therefore with the purely hæmatological side of the subject.

Virchow designated by the name "Leucocytosis," a transient increase in the number of the leucocytes in the blood; and taught that it occurred in many physiological and pathological conditions. In the period that followed particular attention was paid to the leucocytosis in infectious diseases, and to the investigators of the last 15 years in this province we owe very important conclusions as to the **biological meaning** of this symptom. Above all Metschnikoff has done pioneer service in this direction by his theory of phagocytes, and though his theory has been shaken in many essential points, yet it has exercised a stimulating and fruitful influence on the whole field of investigation.

To sketch Metschnikoff's doctrine in a few strokes is only possible by a paraphrase of the very pregnant words "Phagocytes, digestive cells." These words express the view, that the leucocytes defend the organism against bacteria by imprisoning them by the aid of their pseudo-podia, taking them up into their substance, and so depriving them of the power of external influence. The issue of an infectious disease would chiefly depend on whether the number of leucocytes in the blood is sufficient for this purpose.

This engaging theory of Metschnikoff has undergone important limitations as the result of further investigation. Denys, Buchner, Martin Hahn, Goldscheider and Jacob, Löwy and Richter, and many others have demonstrated, that the most important weapon of the leucocytes is not the mechanical one of their pseudopodia, but their chemical products ("Alexine," Bucher). By the aid of bactericidal or antitoxic substances which they secrete, they neutralise the toxines produced by the bacteria, and thus render the foe harmless by destroying his weapon of offence, even if they do not exterminate him.

An explanation of the almost constant increase of the leucocytes of the blood in bacterial diseases is given by the chemiotactic as well as by the phagocytic theory of leucocytosis. The principle of chemiotaxis discovered by Pfeffer asserts that bacteria, or rather their metabolic products, are able to attract by chemical stimulus the cells stored up in the blood-forming organs ("positive chemiotaxis"). In the cases in which a diminution of the leucocytes in the blood is found, it is the result of a repulsion of the leucocytes by the bodies mentioned, negative chemiotaxis.

As the experimental investigation of leucocytosis was carried further, it was found that leucocytosis, quite similar to that occurring in infectious diseases, could also be brought about by the injection of various chemical substances (bacterio-proteins, albumoses, organic extracts and so forth); and it became evident that the explanation of the process by chemiotaxis must be supplemented in many respects. Löwit for instance found that when substances of this kind are injected, two different stages can be distinguished in the behaviour of the leucocytes. First came a stage in which they were diminished ("leukopenia," Löwit) and in such a way that only the polynuclear cells were concerned in the diminution, whilst the number of the lymphocytes was unchanged. After this came the phase of increase of the white blood corpuscles; and here too exclusively of the polynuclear cells; the polynuclear leucocytosis. This behaviour seemed to indicate that during the first period a destruction of white blood corpuscles brought about by the foreign substances took place, and that it was only the dissolved products of the latter which caused the emigration of fresh leucocytes by chemiotaxis. But new objections were raised against this view. Goldscheider and Jacob, in particular, shewed by exact experiments that the transient leukopenia of the blood was not true but merely apparent; and was caused by an altered distribution of the white blood corpuscles within the vascular system. For whilst in the peripheral vessels from which the blood for investigation was usually obtained, there was in fact a diminution of the leucocytes, "hypoleucocytosis," in the capillaries of the internal organs, especially of the lungs, a marked increase of the leucocytes, "hyperleucocytosis," was found.

There are other objections to the great importance that Löwit has given to leukopenia. *A priori* it is quite incomprehensible that the various substances, which in the fundamental test-tube experiment are able to exercise a distinct chemiotactic influence on the leucocytes, should under other circumstances need the intervention of the products of decomposition of the white blood corpuscles. Moreover clinical experince speaks in general against Löwit's theory. For in infectious diseases hyperleucocytosis is very common; and a transient leukopenia is equally rare.

This contradiction to the experimental results obtained by Löwit is easily explained when one reflects how different from the natural processes of disease are the circumstances of experiment. In this case the animal is by intravenous injection flooded at once with the morbid substance, and a violent acute reaction of the vascular and blood systems is the natural consequence. In natural infection, insidious and increasing amounts of poison come quite gradually into play, and for this reason, perhaps, hypoleucocytosis in the normal course of infectious diseases is much rarer than in the brusque conditions of experiment.

Upon the clinical importance of leucocytosis, particularly for the infectious diseases and their various stages, an enormous mass of observations has accumulated. Selecting pneumonia as the best studied example, in the typical course of this disease the constant occurrence of leucocytosis is undisputed; the increase usually continues up to the crisis, and then gives place to a diminution of the leucocytes until a sub-normal number is reached.

Of special importance are the observations on an absence of leucocytosis in particularly severe or lethally ending cases (Kikodse, Sadler, v. Jaksch, Tschistowitch, Türk and others).

In many other diseases as well, the observation has been made that hyperleucocytosis as a rule is only absent in specially severe, or in some way atypical cases. Several observers (Löwy and Richter, M. Hahn, Jacob), have been able to demonstrate experimentally for various infections, that artificial hyperleucocytosis influences the course of an artificial infection most favourably. The question, in what way does this process contribute to the protection of the body, is at the present time under discussion, and introduces the most difficult problems of biology.

---

The **morphological character of leucocytosis** is certainly not simple, and we must sharply separate various groups, according to the kind of leucocyte increased.

The most important consideration is, whether cells capable of spontaneous movement, and of active emigration into the blood, are increased (" **active leucocytosis** "); or whether the number of those cells is raised, to which an independent mobility cannot be ascribed, which therefore are only passively washed into the blood-stream by mechanical forces (" **passive leucocytosis** ").

The passive form of leucocytosis corresponds to the different kinds of lymphæmia, including that of leukæmia. In the section on the lymphatic glands, we have established this view in detail, and we have particularly insisted that a suppuration, consisting of lymph cells, does not occur.

In sharp contrast to this form there are for every specific kind of active leucocytosis, analogous products of inflammation (pus, exudations), composed of the same kind of cell.

We divide active leucocytosis into the following groups :

(α)  polynuclear leucocytoses:

1.  polynuclear neutrophil leucocytosis,

2.  polynuclear eosinophil leucocytosis;

(β)  mixed leucocytoses in which the granulated mononuclear elements take part; "myelæmia."

## α. 1.  Polynuclear neutrophil leucocytosis,

is the most frequent of all forms of active leucocytoses.

Virchow, the discoverer of leucocytosis, advocated the view, that it resulted from an increased stimulation of the lymph glands. The stimulation of the lymph glands consists in "that they are engaged in an increased formation of cells, that their follicles enlarge, and after a time contain many more cells than before." The swelling of the lymphatic glands has as a consequence an increase of the lymph corpuscles in the lymph, and through this an increase again of the colourless blood corpuscles.

This standpoint had to be abandoned, when Ehrlich shewed that it is chiefly the emigration of the polynuclear neutrophil cells, which brings about leucocytosis. Exact figures on this point were first given by Einhorn, who worked under Ehrlich, and were later generally confirmed. Corresponding with the increase of neutrophil blood corpuscles alone, there is always a relative decrease of lymphocytes, often to $2\,^{\circ}/_{\circ}$ and even lower. It must here be borne in mind, that the percentage of the lymph cells may be much diminished, without change in their absolute number. It has however been conclusively demonstrated that occasionally in polynuclear leucocytosis, the absolute number of the lymphocytes may decrease. Einhorn had already described a case of this kind, and recently Türk has for the first time established the fact by an abundance of numerical estimations[1].

The eosinophil cells are as a rule diminished in ordinary polynuclear leucocytosis, as Erhlich had already mentioned in his first communication. The diminution is often considerable, often indeed absolute.

A few diseases shew, besides the neutrophil leucocytosis, an increase of the eosinophils as well, as we shall describe in detail in the next section.

Polynuclear neutrophil leucocytosis—leucocytosis κατ' ἐξοχὴν—may be divided into several groups according to their clinical occurrence. We distinguish:

## A.    physiological leucocytosis,

which appears in health as an expression of changes in the physiological state. To this group belongs the leucocytosis of digestion, the leucocytosis from bodily exertion (Schumburg and Zuntz) or from cold baths, and further the leucocytosis of pregnancy.

## B.    pathological leucocytosis.

1. The increase of polynuclear cells occurring in infectious processes, often called inflammatory, after the principle "*a potiori fit denominatio*." The majority of febrile infectious diseases, pneumonia, erysipelas, diphtheria, septic conditions of the most varied ætiology, parotitis, acute articular rheumatism, etc. are accompanied by a leucocytosis of greater or less extent. In this connection uncomplicated typhoid fever and measles

---

[1] Naturally an ordinary leucocytosis may be combined with a lymph-æmia. We have already mentioned elsewhere (see page 102) that in the leucocytosis of digestion or of diseases of the intestine in children, such a coincidence occurs.

occupy a peculiar position. In them the absolute number of white blood corpuscles is diminished, and chiefly at the expense of the polynuclear neutrophil cells.

For the details we have quoted, and for the course and variations of leucocytosis in infectious diseases we refer to the thorough monograph of Türk. Of Türk's observations we will mention only that in the final stage of the process of leucocytosis, which occurs at the time of the crisis in diseases which run their course critically, mononuclear neutrophil cells and stimulation forms as well often make their appearance in the blood. In still later stages, in which the blood has once more a nearly normal composition, a moderate increase of the eosinophils—gradually waxing and again waning—is very frequently found (Zappert and others). Stiénon, who has likewise devoted special researches to the occurrence of leucocytosis in infectious diseases, shews this point very well in his curves.

2. Toxic leucocytosis occurring in intoxications with the so-called blood poisons. This important group has not yet received adequate treatment in the literature. In general the majority of blood poisons, potassium chlorate, the derivatives of phenyl hydrazin, pyrodin, phenacetin call forth even in man a considerable increase of the leucocytes besides the destruction of the red blood corpuscles. This has been observed experimentally by Rieder.

We observed marked increase of the white blood corpuscles after poisoning from arsenurietted hydrogen, from potassium chlorate, further in a fatally ending case of hæmoglobinuria (sulphonal poisoning?) as well as after protracted chloroform narcosis.

3. The leucocytosis which accompanies acute and chronic anæmic conditions, especially posthæmorrhagic.

4. Cachectic leucocytosis in malignant tumours, phthisis, etc.[1]

To enter here more precisely into the special clinical importance of blood investigation in different forms of disease would lead us too far, and we refer for this subject to the excellent and thorough monograph on leucocytosis by Rieder and to the papers of Zappert and Türk. In this place we will only touch on the most weighty points.

α. The importance for differential diagnosis of the leukopenic blood condition in typhoid fever as compared with other infectious diseases, and in measles as against scarlet fever.

β. The prognostic importance of the enumeration of the white blood corpuscles. Thus for example the absence of leucocytosis influences the prognosis of pneumonia unfavourably (Kikodse and others); and the appearance of numerous myelocytes in diphtheria is ominous, as demonstrated by C. S. Engel (see page 78).

---

Finally, we may dismiss in a few words the origin of **polynuclear neutrophil leucocytosis,** and refer to

[1] The so-called agony leucocytosis we do not regard as a true leucocytosis, but only as the expression of a stoppage of the circulation caused by that condition. This produces an accumulation of the white corpuscles on the vessel walls, especially in the peripheral parts of the body which are as a rule used for clinical investigation. A leucocytosis is thus simulated.

what has been said in another place on the function of the bone-marrow.

In agreement with Kurloff's researches, Ehrlich formulated ("On severe anæmic conditions" 1892) his views on this subject as follows: "The bone-marrow is a breeding place in which polynuclear cells are produced in large numbers from mononuclear pre-existing forms. These polynuclear cells possess above all other elements the power of emigration. So soon as chemiotactic substances circulate in the blood, which attract the white elements, this power comes into play. This readily explains the rapid and sudden appearance of large numbers of leucocytes, which so many substances bring about, and particularly the bacterio-proteins, recognised by Buchner as leucocytic stimuli. I regard leucocytosis therefore, in agreement with Kurloff, as a function of the bone-marrow."

Of great theoretical interest is the contrast between eosinophil and neutrophil cells. At the height of ordinary leucocytosis, the number of eosinophil cells is diminished often to disappearance; whilst during its decline they occur in abnormally high numbers. Hence it follows that the eosinophil and neutrophil cells must react towards stimulating substances completely differently, and in a certain sense oppositely[1].

It seems, generally speaking, that the bacterial

[1] It is also of interest to notice the behaviour of the eosinophil cells in the passive form of leucocytosis, lymphæmia. _À priori_ both conditions could be combined. As C. S. Engel has established in the congenital syphilis of children a simultaneous marked increase of lymphocytes and eosinophil cells is found. The lymphocytosis in these cases is probably due to the anatomical changes of the lymph glands, and the eosinophilia to specific chemiotactic attraction.

metabolic products formed in human diseases which are positively chemiotactic for the polynuclear neutrophil cells are negatively chemiotactic for the eosinophils, and *vice versâ*.

The explanation of the individual clinical forms of leucocytosis is self-evident from the above description. The occurrence of physiological and inflammatory leucocytosis is exclusively to be explained by chemiotaxis. In the other forms, however, other factors also come into play, in particular the increased activity of the bone-marrow, or the extensive transformation of fatty to red marrow, causing a large fresh formation of leucocytes.

## α 2. Polynuclear eosinophil leucocytosis. Mast cells.

Our knowledge of eosinophil leucocytosis is still of comparatively recent date. After Ehrlich demonstrated the constant increase of the eosinophil cells in leukæmia a considerable time elapsed before an eosinophilia was found in other diseases, an eosinophilia however that differs in its essential traits from the leukæmic type. To Friedrich Müller we owe the first researches in this direction, at whose suggestion Gollasch investigated the blood of persons suffering from asthma; in which he was able to demonstrate a considerable increase of the eosinophil cells. This was followed by the researches of H. F. Müller and Rieder, who discovered the frequency of eosinophilia in children, and its presence in chronic splenic tumours; further by the well-known work of Ed. Neusser, who observed a quite astounding increase of the oxyphil elements in pemphigus, and by the almost simultaneous analogous observations of Canon in chronic skin diseases. From amongst the flood of further papers upon this condition we will only mention the comprehensive account of the subject by Zappert.

By eosinophilia we understand an increase only of the polynuclear eosinophil cells in the blood. Confusion of this form of leucocytosis with leukæmia is quite impossible, because a good number of characteristic signs are necessary for the diagnosis of the latter, as we shall have to explain in the next section. The presence of mononuclear eosinophil cells in the blood should not be regarded, as is the case in many quarters, as an absolute proof of leukæmia, for they are also found in isolated cases of ordinary leucocytosis.

The increase of eosinophil cells is not always relative, but may be absolute. The relative number, normally 2 to 4% of all leucocytes, rises in eosinophilia to 10, 20, 30% and over; in a case described by Grawitz 90% indeed was found. The thorough researches of Zappert, carried out on moist preparations by a suitable method, are particularly instructive with regard to their absolute number. As the lowest normal value he gives 50—100 eosinophil cells per mm.$^3$, as mean value 100 to 200, as a high normal value 200—250. The highest absolute number he has ever found was 29,000 per mm.$^3$ in leukæmia, the highest number in simple eosinophil leucocytosis 4800 (in a case of pemphigus). Reinbach indeed once found about 60,000 eosinophil cells per mm.$^3$ in a case of lymphosarcoma of the neck with metastases in the bone-marrow.

Polynuclear eosinophil leucocytosis, apart from the form observed in healthy children, occurs in varied conditions, and for comprehensiveness we divide them into several groups.  We distinguish eosinophilia:

1.  In bronchial asthma.  Increase of the eosinophil cells of the blood, often considerable, amounting to 10 and 20 % and more has been regularly found, first by Gollasch, later by many other observers.  (For the special clinical course of the eosinophilia in asthma see below.)

2.  In pemphigus.  Neusser first recorded that an extraordinarily great, indeed a specific eosinophilia was found in many cases of pemphigus.  This interesting observation has been confirmed on many sides, in particular by Zappert, who once observed 4800 oxyphil per mm.[3]

3.  In acute and chronic skin-diseases.  Canon was the first to notice that in a fairly large number of skin-diseases, especially in prurigo and psoriasis, the eosinophil cells are increased up to 17 %.  The observation of Canon is worthy of attention, that the increase of the eosinophils is connected with the degree of extension of the disease, rather than with its nature or local intensity.  In a case of acute widely distributed urticaria, A. Lazarus found the eosinophils increased to 60 % of the leucocytes, a number which after the course of a few days again sank to normal.

4.  In helminthiasis.  The first observations on the occurrence of eosinophilia in helminthiasis we owe to Müller and Rieder, who obtained fairly high values (8·2 and 9·7 %) in two men suffering from Ankylostomum duodenale.  Shortly afterwards Zappert stated that he had found a considerable increase of the eosinophil cells in the blood, reaching 17 % in two cases of the same

disease; at the same time he demonstrated Charcot's crystals in the fæces. In a third case of Ankylostomiasis Zappert found no increase of eosinophil cells in the blood, nor the crystals in the fæces. Almost simultaneously, Siege made similar observations.

For a detailed working out of this important branch we are greatly indebted to Leichtenstern. Under his direction Bücklers established the interesting fact that Ankylostomiasis in its relation to eosinophilia does not occupy a special place in diseases caused by worms. All kinds of Helminthides, from the harmless Oxyuris to the pernicious Ankylostoma, may bring about an increase of the eosinophil cells in the blood, often to an enormous extent[1]. Bücklers reports an observation of 16% eosinophils in Oxyurides, of 19% in Ascarides; and Prof. Leichtenstern, as we learn from a private communication, has quite recently found 72% eosinophil cells in a case of Ankylostomiasis, and 34% in a case of Tænia mediocanellata.

It is well worthy of note that Leichtenstern was able to observe numerous eosinophil cells in the blood in those cases where Charcot's crystals were abundantly contained in the fæces. Since eosinophil cells and Charcot's crystals have elsewhere been observed to be interconnected phenomena (for example in bronchial asthma, in nasal polypi, in myelæmic blood and bone-marrow) one must fall in with Leichtenstern's supposition that eosinophil cells ought also to be found in the intestinal mucus in cases of Ankylostomiasis. Positive observations on this point as yet are wanting.

[1] In his monograph on Bothriocephalus anæmia Schauman, with reference to the behaviour of the eosinophil cells, states that he has found them in but few cases of this disease.

T. R. Brown, who worked under direction of Thayer, has lately communicated the interesting observation that in trichinosis there is constantly an extraordinary relative increase in the oxyphil leucocytes in the blood, up to 68 %. The absolute figures were also much raised, and attained values (20,400 for example) which are by no means frequent even in leukæmia.

Brown regards this astonishing phenomenon as pathognomic for trichinosis, so much so, that in a case that was clinically obscure, he made, from the marked eosinophilia, the diagnosis of trichinosis which was later fully confirmed.

5. Post-febrile form of eosinophilia (after the termination of various infectious diseases). In the section on polynuclear neutrophil leucocytosis we have already mentioned that at the height of most of the acute infectious diseases, with the single exception of scarlet fever, the eosinophils undergo a relative decrease and may even entirely disappear. In the post-febrile period, however, abnormally high values for the eosinophil cells are often found, or even a well-marked eosinophil leucocytosis, which generally attains but moderate degree. Türk for example in pneumonia found a post-critical eosinophilia of $5.67$ % (430 absolute), after acute articular rheumatism $9.37$ % (970 absolute); Zappert in malaria, one day after the last attack $20.34$ % (1486 per mm.[3]).

The eosinophilia observed as the result of tuberculin injections, we include, in agreement with Zappert, in the group of post-febrile leucocytosis. For it appears only after considerable rises of temperature. During the real reaction period the number of eosinophil cells sinks, and only goes up again after the termination of the fever. The rise may be very considerable. In one case of

Zappert's the number of the oxyphils increased to 26·9 %; in another of his cases the highest absolute figure formed after tuberculin injections was 3220 per mm.[3] In a case of Grawitz' the eosinophilia was quite extraordinary. The most marked changes in the blood occurred some three weeks after cessation of the tuberculin injections, of which eight altogether (from 5 mg. to 38 mg.) were given. Investigation shewed 4,000,000 red blood corpuscles per mm.[3], 45,000 white. Amongst the latter there were ten eosinophils to one non-eosinophil. The total number of eosinophil cells amounted to some 41,000 per mm.[3], whilst the other cells as a whole made up some 4000. Inasmuch as the latter contained polynuclears, lymphocytes and other forms, it follows that in this case the polynuclear neutrophils must have been very much decreased, not only relatively but also absolutely; so that this case represents precisely the contrary condition to ordinary leucocytosis and the infectious form in particular.

6. In malignant tumours. In the cachexia from tumours an increase of the eosinophil cells has been observed by various authors. It is however of moderate degree and does not exceed 7—10 %. Out of 40 decided cases Reinbach found the eosinophils increased only in four, in a case of sarcoma of the forearm he found 7·8 %; of the thigh 8·4 %; malignant tumour of the abdomen 11·6 %. Besides these he describes a case of lymphosarcoma of the neck with metastases in the bone-marrow, in which an unexampled increase of the white blood corpuscles, and especially of the eosinophil cells was found. The absolute number of the latter amounted on one day to some 60,000! This is an increase of 300 fold the normal, which apart from leukæmia has doubtless never before been found.

7. Compensatory eosinophilia (after exclusion of the spleen). We have entered in detail into this form in the chapter on splenic function; and have there already mentioned that the increase of the eosinophils found in chronic splenic tumours by Rieder, Weiss and others, must also be referred to the exclusion of the splenic function.

8. Medicinal eosinophilia. Under this group occurs only a single observation of v. Noorden's, who observed the appearance of an eosinophilia up to 9 % in two chlorotic girls after internal administration of camphor. In other patients this occurrence did not repeat itself. But probably researches specially directed to this province of pharmacology would bring to our knowledge many interesting facts.

On the origin of **polynuclear eosinophil leuco-cytosis** authors have put forward various theories, which we will here critically discuss in succession.

An experiment frequently quoted as explanatory is that of Müller and Rieder's; these authors do not derive the eosinophil cells of the blood from the bone-marrow, but assume, as very probable, that the finely granular cells grow into eosinophils within the blood-stream. This developmental process seems very im-probable for many reasons. Since the polynuclear cells circulating in the blood are all under the same conditions of nutrition, it is à priori inconceivable why only a relatively small portion of them should undergo the transformation in question. And it is quite inex-plicable why in infectious leucocytosis, where the number of the polynuclears is increased so enormously, their ripening to the eosinophils should remain completely interrupted.

But the fact, that a transition from neutrophil to oxyphil cells has never really been observed in the blood, is decisive evidence against the hypothesis of Müller and Rieder. Were the hypothesis true, transitional stages ought to be found with ease in every sample of normal blood. Rieder and Müller themselves are unable to bring forward any positive result of this kind, else they would hardly have been contented to fall back on the authority of Max Schultze, who professed to shew the transitional forms between the finely and coarsely granular leucocytes in the circulating blood. The authority of Max Schultze in morphological questions stands high, and very rightly; but one ought not to rely upon it for support in problems that are really histo-chemical, and which should be solved by their appropriate methods.

As a logical consequence of their view, and in decided opposition to Ehrlich, Müller and Rieder assume that the eosinophil cells of the bone-marrow "are far rather the expression of a storage than of a fresh formation there. The bone-marrow therefore should be regarded in reference to the coarsely granular cells of the blood more as a storage depôt, where these cells serve other purposes, which for the present cannot be more closely defined."

The chief reason for this assumption, these authors see in the fact, that the majority of the eosinophils in the bone-marrow are mononuclear, whilst those of normal blood possess a polymorphous nucleus. Müller and Rieder should themselves have raised the obvious objection that the same holds good for the nucleus of the neutrophils. They would then have seen the fault in their theory; for according to it the most important blood preparing organ constitutes as it were, not the cradle of the blood cells, but their grave. The simplest and readiest explanation, based too upon histological observation, is surely this: that the mononuclear eosinophil cells grow into polynuclear in the bone-marrow, but that the latter only reach the blood by means of their power of emigration. As this view has been accepted by the great majority of authors since Ehrlich's paper " On severe anæmic conditions," we believe we may content ourselves with the above objections to the Müller-Rieder theory, although it has even quite recently found supporters (*e.g.* B. Lenhartz). H. F. Müller moreover in his paper on bronchial asthma (1893) takes a position different from his earlier, and approaching that of Ehrlich.

In considering the production of polynuclear eosinophilia we may best start from an experiment of E. Neusser's. Neusser found in a pemphigus patient, whose blood shewed a considerable increase of the eosinophils, that the contents of the pemphigus bulla consisted almost entirely of eosinophil cells. Neusser now produced a non-specific inflammatory bulla in the skin by a vesicant, and found that the cellular elements in it were exclusively the polynuclear neutrophil concerned in all ordinary inflammations.

Exactly analogous conditions, occurring spontaneously, have been demonstrated by Leredde and Perrin in the so-called Dühring's disease. The bullæ which appear in this dermatosis contain, so long as their contents are clear, chiefly polynuclear eosinophil cells. In a later stage, as is usually the case, bacteria effect an entrance into the bullæ, which now become filled with neutrophils.

According to modern views on suppuration, the experiment of Neusser and the observation of Leredde and Perrin can only be explained by the hypothesis, that the eosinophil and neutrophil cells, as we have already several times mentioned, are of different chemiotactic irritability. Hence the eosinophil cells only emigrate to those parts where a specific stimulating substance is present. From this point of view experiments and clinical observations known up to the present on eosinophilia may be readily explained. Neusser's experiment for instance may be explained in the following way. In the pemphigus bullæ a substance is present that chemiotactically attracts the eosinophils. Hence the cells normally contained in the blood emigrate into them, and produce the picture of an eosinophilous suppuration. Should the disease assume from the first a localised distribution only, the essential feature of the process is excluded. A totally different appearance, however, is produced when the disease has attacked large areas. Under these circumstances large amounts of the specific active agent reach the blood-stream by absorption and diffusion. Here it exercises a strong chemiotactic influence on the physiological storage depôt of the eosinophils, the bone-marrow; leading to an increase of the eosinophils of the blood to a greater or less degree. The bone-marrow, according to general biological laws, is by the increased emigration now further stimulated to a fresh production, and during a protracted illness can hence keep up the eosinophilia.

In this way other clinical observations may be explained. Gollasch has found that the sputum of asthmatic patients contains, in addition to Charcot-Leyden's crystals, eosinophil cells only. One must therefore assume that within the bronchial tree there exists material which attracts the eosinophils. This supposition is also supported by the close connection that obtains, according to many observations, between the severity of the disease and the eosinophilia. Thus v. Noorden records that the eosinophil cells are more numerous about the time of an attack. They accumulated in especially large numbers after attacks had rapidly occurred several days in succession. That the increase of the eosinophil cells in this instance is directly connected with the attacks, and is not the expression of a permanent constitutional anomaly, is shewn by a case in which v. Noorden found $25\,^0/_0$ eosinophils during the attack, and a few days later could only observe one example in twelve cover-slip preparations : a diminution therefore of this group of cells.

The observations of Canon in skin-diseases are quite similar, for he shewed that the extension of the disease determines the degree of eosinophilia more than its intensity. And it is the former factor which directly determines the quantities of the specific agent that pass into the blood.

To the Müller-Rieder hypothesis, and the chemiotactic theory of eosinophil leucocytosis a third has lately been added, which may be shortly called the hypothesis of the local origin of the eosinophil cells. A. Schmidt has, with special reference to asthma, raised the question "whether in the extensive production of eosinophil cells in asthma, local production in the air passages is not more probable than origin from the blood. One may well regard the increase of the eosinophil cells in the blood of an asthmatic as secondary." This view, which has also been advocated by other authors, rests more particularly on the following facts and considerations :

　　1.　That in various diseases of the nose, especially in

mucous polypi and hyperplasia of the mucous membrane (Leyden, Benno Lewy and others), a great accumulation of eosinophil cells is found in these tissues, whilst they are apparently not increased in the blood. This objection is easily laid aside from the chemiotactic point of view. For if in the places in question substances are present which act chemiotactically on the eosinophil leucocytes, in the course of time marked accumulation must occur, without an increase of their number in the blood. One might as well conclude from Neumann's experiment in lymphatic leukæmia, for example, where the artificial suppuration consisted only of polynuclear neutrophil cells, that the polynuclear cells were formed in the tissue, since in the blood they were present in very small percentage. For in this case too the same incongruity between the blood and the particular tissue exists.

2.  Adolph Schmidt has urged the converse argument. He shewed that in the sputum of patients with myelogenic leukæmia no more eosinophil cells were present than are commonly to be found in the bronchial secretion, although the blood was unusually rich in eosinophil cells. In our opinion however this observation does not support the hypothesis of local origin, but on the contrary is clear evidence that not the larger or smaller number of eosinophil cells in the blood decides their emigration, but the presence of specifically active chemical stimuli. For we know from our observations on leucocytosis in infectious diseases that the bacterial stimulating substances act on the eosinophil cells rather in a negative than in a positive sense. And if ordinary sputum is not rich in eosinophils in spite of a marked eosinophilia of the blood, this only corresponds to our experience in general. Indeed, this phenomenon is quite similar to Neusser's pemphigus

experiment, where the specific foci of disease shewed an eosinophilia, whilst abscesses produced artificially, on the contrary, only neutrophil cells. Finally we may employ, to support our view, another analogous experiment of Schmidt himself. He found numerous eosinophil cells in the sputum of an asthmatic patient, but only neutrophil cells in an artificially produced suppuration of the skin.

Thus we see that the chief reasons brought forward by the supporters of the theory of local origin are not proof against the most obvious objections that can be raised from the chemiotactic standpoint. Moreover, neither histological nor experimental proof has been given for this theory in spite of numerous investigations in this direction. All the same, it should not be out of place to explain the possibilities that are given for a local origin of the eosinophil cells. First, the eosinophil cells might be the result of a progressive metamorphosis of the normal tissue cells. That such a process is possible, is proved by the local origin of the mast cells. These may arise, as Ehrlich and his school have always assumed, by transformation of pre-existing connective tissue cells[1]; but that the same holds good for the eosinophil cells as well, has nowise as yet been proved. Secondly, it is conceivable, that isolated eosinophil cells, pre-existing in the tissues, should rapidly multiply, and so produce the local accumulation only. Numerous mitoses could be considered an adequate proof of this process. But so far no figures of nuclear division have been observed; indeed A. Schmidt,

[1] This view has lately received striking confirmation from the interesting experiment of Baümer, who produced on himself by means of continued stimulation with *Urticaria ureus* a considerable increase in four days of the mast cells in the irritated portions of the skin.

who has directed special experiments thereto from the standpoint of his theory, has found them entirely absent.

As a third possibility for the local origin of the eosinophil cells, their direct descent from neutrophil cells is conceivable, and is by many regarded as a kind of ripening. This assumption nevertheless must be described as unsound, since the necessary condition of its foundation, namely the observation of corresponding transitional stages, has not so far been fulfilled.

By the inductive method then we conclude that a local origin of the eosinophil cells can hardly come under discussion. And this conclusion is strengthened by comparison with the behaviour of the mast cells, which are related to the eosinophils in many points, and only differ from them essentially in the nature of their granulation. The mast cells too, like the eosinophils, form a normal constituent of the bone-marrow, and occur regularly besides in normal blood, though in very small number—according to Canon they amount to 0·28% of the leucocytes. We know that the mast cells are produced in large quantities locally, wherever an over-nutrition of the connective tissue occurs, for instance in chronic diseases of the skin, elephantiasis, brown induration of the lungs. In the case of the mast cells, then, we see the conditions actually realised, which the supporters of the theory of the local origin of the eosinophil cells only assume. We should therefore expect that an increase of mast cells in the blood or in certain inflammatory exudations would be by no means seldom. With this point in mind Ehrlich has subjected the sputum in emphysema and brown induration of the lungs to exact examination for 20 years. Nevertheless he has obtained entirely negative results. The special blood investigations of

Canon have likewise proved to be practically negative. In 22 healthy persons Canon entirely failed to find the mast cells on nine occasions, in the others he found on the average 0·47 %; the highest percentage number obtained was 0·89 %. Only in a few cases of skin disease was a slight increase indicated. The average amounted to 0·58 %, a number, therefore, which is often to be found in healthy individuals. A leucocytosis of mast cells, comparable with the eosinophil or neutrophil forms of leucocytosis, has not been demonstrated in the cases of Canon or other observers. On the other hand, the mast cells undergo a considerable increase in myelogenic leukæmia, in many cases equalling or even exceeding that of the eosinophils. We shall not err in deriving the mast cells of the blood solely from the bone-marrow, on the grounds of this fact; or in conjecturing that their origin is not from the connective tissue, even when they are there excessively increased[1].

We think we have shewn in the preceding paragraphs that the evidence, so far brought forward for a local origin of the eosinophil cells, does not withstand the objections that have been raised. The task now lies before us, to produce positive proof that the accumulations of eosinophil cells in the organs and secretions must be explained by emigration from the blood.

---

[1] That a well-marked basophil leucocytosis has not so far been observed may be thus explained. The substances which attract the mast cells are very rarely produced in the body; much more seldom than the corresponding substances attractive for the eosinophils. In morbid conditions, where substances attracting the mast cells were present, it might be possible to find a suppuration of mast cells, or a mast cell leucocytosis as well. In this connection an observation of Albert Neisser is of the greatest interest. He met with (private communication) one, out of numberless cases of gonorrhœa, in which the purulent secretion consisted entirely of mast cells.

This proof offers great difficulties in as much as we normally find eosinophil cells in many places. Here then we cannot trace a process step by step, but we have to deal with final conditions. Could we observe the genesis of eosinophil cells in organs usually free from them, it would be easier to clear up this question. Up to the present but a single observation on this point is available. Michælis established the interesting fact, that on interrupting lactation in suckling guinea-pigs, in the course of a few days numerous eosinophil cells collect in the mammary glands, but not in the lumen of the canaliculi. The eosinophil cells are further polynuclear, exactly corresponding to those of the blood, and therefore to be regarded as immigrants. We may explain this condition according to modern views as follows. Under certain conditions the mammary gland is capable of an internal secretion, by means of which substances are produced that are specifically chemiotactic for the eosinophil cells. When the external secretion of milk is disturbed, the internal secretion is abnormally increased. The fact too that in Michælis' researches no eosinophil cells passed into the true secretion of the gland may be thus explained[1].

Exactly similar observations have been made on pathological material, first recorded in the brilliant and fundamental work of Goldmann. In a case of malignant lymphoma Goldmann found a considerable accumulation of eosinophil cells within the tumour, and demonstrated anatomically, that it was brought about by an emigration of the cells from the vascular system. Hence Goldmann

[1] Unger has recently published completely analogous observations on the human breast for the mast cells. Under the influence of stagnation of the milk he saw an invasion of the gland tissue by typical mast cells.

concluded that the eosinophil cells pass over into the tissue in question, at the call of certain chemiotactic products. Goldmann, and later Kauter, shewed that these eosinophil cells were not merely due to an ordinary inflammation; for in a large number of other diseases of the lymph glands—particularly the tuberculous, they were entirely absent. Similarly Leredde and Perrin have shewn in their investigations of Dühring's disease, that the eosinophil cells, which are also present in the cutaneous tissue in large numbers, apart from the contents of the bullæ, are due to an emigration from the blood-stream.

Thus it is evident from a number of various facts, that the eosinophil cells found in the tissues are not formed there, but have immigrated from the blood-stream. It naturally often happens that this appearance is not preserved equally distinctly in all cases. For, as has been seen in the ordinary polynuclear leucocytes, the immigrated polynuclear eosinophils may similarly change to mononuclear cells; they may perhaps settle down, and approximate to the character of fixed connective tissue cells. Such appearances may readily give rise to the view that in this case the reverse nuclear metamorphosis has occurred; that is a progressive development from mononuclear eosinophil to polynuclear cells.

In agreement with Goldmann, Jadassohn and H. F. Müller, we believe that the only admissible explanation for the facts mentioned above is that the eosinophil cells obey specific chemiotactic stimuli. By this hypothesis we can easily understand eosinophil leucocytosis, the presence of eosinophil cells in exudations and secretions, and the local accumulation of this kind of cell.

As to the nature of these chemiotactically active

substances, we can so far only surmise. From amongst the clinical phenomena capable of throwing light on this subject we mention once more the fact, that the metabolic products of bacteria repel the eosinophil cells.

The opposed behaviour of eosinophil and neutrophil cells is very well illustrated by a case of Leichtenstern:

"In a very anæmic almost moribund patient with Ankylostomias there were found 72 % eosinophil cells in the blood in 1897. The patient contracted a croupous pneumonia, and in the high febrile period of the disease the number of eosinophils sank to 6—7 %, and rose again after the termination of the pneumonia to 54 %. After removal of the worm the number at once fell to 11 %. In the year 1898 the patient harboured but a very few Ankylostomata; Charcot's crystals were no longer present in the fæces; the number of the eosinophils amounted to 8 %."

The question, what cells produce on their destruction actively chemiotactic substances, is of very great importance; but cannot be answered with the material at present available. The breaking up of ordinary pus cells or lymphocytes does not appear to give rise to any such substances; but there is much evidence that the decomposition products of epithelial and epithelioid cells act chemiotactically. Thus we can explain the frequent occurrence of eosinophilia in all kinds of skin-diseases. Again, in all atrophic conditions of the gastric, intestinal and bronchial mucous membrane there occurs a local accumulation of eosinophil cells; further, this kind of cell is increased in the neighbourhood of carcinoma. Additional support for this view is seen in the fact that in bronchitis and asthma the less the suppurative element of the secretion is developed, the more numerous are the eosinophil cells. An observation of Jadassohn is worthy of mention in this connection. He observed abundant eosinophil cells in foci of lupus after injection of tuberculin. In these foci then, by the destruction of the epithelioid cells brought about by the tuberculin, substances must have been produced which act chemiotactically on the eosinophil cells.

The specific substances are absorbed and reach the blood, and impart to it also the chemiotactic power. The direct cause then of most forms of eosinophilia seems actually to lie in a destruction of tissue, and in the products thus produced.

On the other hand, it cannot be doubted that substances foreign to the organism, circulating in the body, may act chemiotactically on the eosinophil cells[1]. The observations quoted above, of the well-marked eosinophilia in the different forms of Helminthiasis, may here be specially mentioned. The action of the Helminthides was formerly regarded as purely local, but the indications that they act also by the production of poisonous substances continue to increase. Thus Linstow has pointed out that the general typhoid state, and the fatty degeneration of liver and kidneys, that is of organs which the Trichina does not reach, necessitate the assumption of a poisonous substance. And in several varieties of Ankylostoma as well, there is distinct evidence of the production of a poison. We gather from Husemann's article on "animal poisons" (Eulenberg's *Realenencyclopœdie* 1867) that just as Ankylostomum in man produces the well-known severe anæmia, so Ankylostomum trigonocephalum

[1] A very interesting observation of Goldmann's deserves mention here. Goldmann found in preparations of the pancreas of proteus sanguineus, containing parasites, that the eosinophil cells in the neighbourhood of the encapsuled parasites were much increased, whereas they were sought for in vain, in more distant parts.

in the dog, and Ankylostomum perniciosum in the tiger, causes analogous general effects.

Bothriocephalus latus too is now generally accredited with the production of a definite toxic substance; and the common tapeworm even, by no means infrequently brings about injuries to the body which are to be referred to the action of a poison.

So much follows from these observations, that the tapeworms can not only absorb but also can give out substances that are absorbed from the intestine of the host, and are able to bring about distant effects. One expression of these distant actions is, as Leichtenstern insists, the eosinophilia of the blood. We do not think we should assume on the evidence before us, that the substance which attracts the eosinophil cells is identical with the cause of the anæmia. Many observations, the absence, for example, of eosinophilia in Bothriocephalus anæmia (Schauman), render probable the existence of two different functions. In any case the substance causing the eosinophilia is more widely distributed than that to which the anæmic condition is due.

## Leukæmia.

### (" Mixed leucocytosis.")

In spite of the enormous extent of the hæmatological observations of the last decennia, of which a very considerable portion deals with the problem of leukæmia, the literature shews many obscurities and misconceptions, even on important fundamental ideas. This is especially the case with the weighty question of the distinction between various forms of leukæmia.

From the purely clinical standpoint it is usual to

describe a lienal, a lienomedullary, and a pure medullary (myelogenic) form of leukæmia. But the distinguishing characteristics in this classification are crude and purely external, and they find no place in hæmatology.

Neumann first shewed that the lymphoid proliferation in lymphatic anæmia is not confined to the lymph glands, but may extend to the spleen and bone-marrow. These proliferative processes may give rise to a considerable enlargement, for example, of the spleen, without any change in the specific character of the leukæmia, or the condition of the blood. In spite of the splenic tumour we have to deal then with a pure lymphatic leukæmia. In customary clinical language, a case of this kind would be described as lieno-lymphatic leukæmia. The unreliability and incorrectness of this terminology is best illustrated by another form of leukæmic metastasis. In lymphatic leukæmia the liver may swell by lymphomatous growth, to a large tumour, and we ought then to speak of a "hepato-lymphatic" form of leukæmia. This term is by no means so misleading as lieno-lymphatic; for no one would conclude from the former that any liver-cells passed into the blood, whilst the latter implies the idea, that specific splenic cells take part in the blood changes.

Further, the assumption of a pure lienal variety of leukæmia is totally unwarranted from hæmatological investigations. The possibility of a specific blood change, depending solely upon disease of the spleen, appears à priori almost excluded, after what has been said on the physiological participation of the spleen in the formation of the blood.

Pathological data completely confirm this view. Ehrlich at least, in an enormous number of cases, has never once succeeded in confirming the existence of a purely splenic form from the blood examination[1].

The conditions in myelogenic leukæmia are quite similar, for foci of myeloid tissue may appear in the spleen or lymph glands according to the kind of metastasis. As it is the proliferation of the myeloid tissue and not the accompanying swelling of spleen or lymph glands that is specific in the process, the nomenclature "lienomedullary or medullary-lymphatic" leukæmia must also be described as illogical and misleading.

We distinguish then, from the histological standpoint, but two forms of leukæmia:

1. leukæmic processes with proliferation of lymphoid tissue:

**"lymphatic leukæmia"**;

2. leukæmic processes with proliferation of myeloid tissue:

**"myelogenic leukæmia."**

The accompanying clinical phenomena may be indicated by simple unequivocal amplifications, for instance, "lymphatic leukæmia with enlargement of the spleen or of the liver"; "myelogenic leukæmia with enlargement of the lymph glands," &c.

From our present knowledge, which, it may be remarked, is still far from full, we may assume that

[1] A case observed some time back by Ehrlich may here be mentioned as a characteristic example. A woman received a blow in the region of the spleen by a fall from the roof, which gradually led to a marked splenic enlargement. As no other symptoms appeared, the surgeon in charge proposed splenectomy, on the assumption of a pure splenic leukæmia. Examination of the blood, however, shewed a condition fully corresponding with myelogenic leukæmia, and thus prevented surgical interference.

lymphatic and myelogenous leukæmia have quite a
different ætiology. The recent discovery of Löwit should
be decisive on this point, for he demonstrated in myelogenic
leukæmia the presence of forms like plasmodia within the
white blood corpuscles, but was unable to find them in
lymphatic leukæmia.

The necessity of separating lymphatic from myelogenic
leukæmia is further shewn by the fundamental clinical
differences between them.

**Lymphatic leukæmia** falls clinically into two
readily distinguishable forms. In the first place acute
lymphatic leukæmia, characterised by its rapid course,
the small splenic tumour, the tendency to petechiæ and
to the general hæmorrhagic diathesis. By its startling
course this disease has given all observers the impression
of an acute infectious process.

The second form of lymphatic leukæmia is marked off
from the preceding by its chronic, and often very protracted course. The spleen shews its participation in
the disease, as a rule by very considerable enlargement.
We have at present no investigations adequate to decide
whether chronic lymphatic leukæmia represents a single
disease, or should be etiologically subdivided. Hæmato-
logically, all lymphatic leukæmias are characterised by a
great preponderance of lymph cells, in particular of the
larger varieties. It should here be expressly mentioned,
that richness of the blood in large lymph cells, is by no
means characteristic of the acute form of leukæmia, for
chronic, very slowly progressing cases shew the same
condition. Thus in a case of this kind under observation
in Gerhardt's wards, all observers (Grawitz, v. Noorden,
Ehrlich) found the large cells during its whole course.
In agreement with our remarks elsewhere (see p. 104), we

assume with regard to the origin of lymphatic leukæmia, that the increase of the lymph cells is brought about by a passive inflow into the blood; and not by an active emigration from chemical stimuli.

**Myelogenic leukæmia** presents a picture that is different in every particular. In former years the distinction between myelogenic leukæmia and simple leucocytosis offered great difficulties. These conditions were regarded as different stages of one and the same pathological process, and when the proportion of white to red corpuscles exceeded a certain limit (1 : 50) it was said that leucocytosis ceased, and leukæmia began. By the aid of the analytic colour methods the fundamental difference between the two conditions was first disclosed. Leucocytosis is now recognised to be chiefly an increase of the normal polynuclear neutrophil leucocytes; whereas myelogenic leukæmia brings elements into the blood that are abnormal. The cells here introduced are so characteristic as to render the diagnosis of leukæmia possible, even in the very rare cases where the total number of the white blood corpuscles is not to any extent increased. The best example of which we are aware is a case observed by v. Noorden, in which the proportion of white to red was only 1 : 200.

Although the blood picture of myelogenic leukæmia has been so clearly drawn by Ehrlich, misconceptions and obscurities still occur in the literature. And they are due to great errors in observation. It has for instance happened that unskilled observers have regarded and worked up cases of lymphatic leukæmia as myelogenic. The apparent deviations discovered in this manner are copied, as specially remarkable, from one book to another. Through insufficient mastery of the staining method, the characteristic and diagnostically decisive elements (neutrophil myelocytes for example) are frequently mistaken. A further source productive of misconceptions lies in the circumstance that the typical leukæmic condition of the blood may essentially change under the influences of intercurrent diseases. Thus the intrusion of a leucocytosis, brought about by secondary infection, is able to obliterate more or less the specific character of the blood. Such conditions must naturally be considered apart, and should not be used to overthrow the general characteristics of the picture. No one surely would deny the diagnostic value of glycosuria for diabetes, because in conditions of inanition, for instance, the sugar of a diabetic may completely vanish, although the disease continues. And one does not deny the diagnostic value of the splenic tumour in typhoid fever, because the enlargement of the spleen may occasionally subside, under the influence of an intestinal hæmorrhage.

From these considerations it is obviously necessary to derive the description of leukæmic blood from pure uncomplicated cases; and to construct it with the aid of standard methods. In this manner a type is obtained so characteristic, as to render diagnosis absolutely certain from the blood alone.

It is needful here to emphasise this hundred-fold repeated experience with special distinctness, for some recent authors do not even yet allow the full diagnostic importance of the blood examination. v. Limbeck says in the latest edition of his clinical *Pathology of the Blood*, "That one should not regard the blood changes as an invariably reliable diagnostic resource in myelogenic leukæmia; and that the diagnosis of leukæmia should

not rest on the presence or significance of one or more
cells. Not only the general features of the case, but
the blood condition as well should be considered." To
these remarks the objection must be made that up
to the present no serious hæmatologist will have had
to diagnose a leukæmic disease principally "from the
presence of one or more cells." In the work of Ehrlich
and his pupils at least, it has always been shewn
that the character of a leukæmic condition is only
settled by a concurrence of a large number of single
symptoms, of which each one is indispensable for the
diagnosis, and which taken together are absolutely conclusive. With these premisses it is indisputable that
the microscopic examination of the blood alone
on dry preparations, without the assistance of
any other clinical method, can decide whether
a patient suffers from leukæmia, and whether
it belongs to the lymphatic or myelogenic
variety.

The microscopic picture of myelogenic leukæmia, disregarding the almost constant increase of the
white blood corpuscles, has a varied, highly inconstant
character. This arises from the co-operation of several
anomalies, namely:

A. that in addition to the polynuclear cells,
their early stages, the mononuclear granulated
corpuscles likewise circulate in the blood;

B. that all three types of granulated cells,
the neutrophil, eosinophil, and mast cells par-
ticipate in the increase of the white blood
corpuscles;

C. that atypical cell-forms appear, *e.g.* dwarf

forms of all the kinds of white corpuscles; and further mitotic nuclear figures;

D. that the blood always contains nucleated red blood corpuscles, often in great numbers.

1. We begin with the discussion of the mononuclear neutrophil cells, Ehrlich's "myelocytes." They are present so abundantly in the blood of medullary leukæmia as to impart to the whole picture a predominantly mononuclear character. As we have frequently mentioned, myelocytes occur normally only in the bone-marrow, not in the circulating blood. Their eminent importance for the diagnosis of myelogenic leukæmia, where they have been regularly found by the best observers, is in no way diminished by their transitory appearance in a few other conditions (see pages 77, 78). Though they have been occasionally found, according to Türk's investigations, in the critical period of pneumonia as parts of a general leucocytosis, the danger of confusion with leukæmic blood changes is non-existent. This is guarded against by (1) the much smaller increase of the white cells; (2) the diminution of the eosinophil and mast cells; (3) the fact, that the myelocytes of leukæmic blood are nearly always considerably larger; (4) the preponderating polynuclear character of the leucocytosis, which is not effaced by the small percentage amount of myelocytes (at most $12\,^o/_o$): (5) the incomparably smaller absolute number of myelocytes. In the most pronounced case of Türk's, for example, in which the percentage number of myelocytes amounted to $11\cdot9$, calculation of their absolute number gives at most 1000 myelocytes per mm.[3] This is a figure which bears no comparison with that obtaining in leukæmia, where 50,000—100,000 myelocytes per mm.[3] and over occur in cases that are in no way extreme.

2. The mononuclear eosinophil cells. Before the introduction of the staining method, Mosler had described large, coarsely granulated cells, "marrow cells," as characteristic for myelogenic leukæmia. These are to be regarded as for the most part identical with the mononuclear eosinophil cells, noticed by Müller and Rieder as peculiar, and aptly described by them as the eosinophil analogues of the preceding group. They appear as large elements with oval, feebly staining nucleus. Undeniably a valuable sign of leukæmia, they are not nearly so important as the mononuclear neutrophil cells, as follows from the numerical superiority of the latter. To regard the presence of "eosinophil myelocytes" as absolute proof of the existence of a leukæmia is inadmissible, since they are occasionally present in small numbers in other diseases.

3. The absolute increase of the eosinophil cells. In his first paper on leukæmia, Ehrlich stated that the absolute number of polynuclear eosinophils is always much increased in myelogenic leukæmia. This assertion of Ehrlich has been received under some protest ; v. Limbeck in his text-book even speaks of an "alleged" increase of the eosinophil cells. The well-known work of Müller and Rieder has more particularly given rise to this opposition, and thrown doubt on the diagnostic importance of the eosinophil cells. These authors however base their contradiction on false premises.

For Ehrlich did not speak of a rise of the percentage of the eosinophil cells, but only of an increase in their absolute number. If in a case of leukæmia only the normal percentage number of eosinophils is found, it indicates, all the same, a great absolute increase ; and Müller and Rieder would themselves have fully confirmed

Ehrlich's statement, had they only calculated the absolute figures in a few of their cases. Selecting from the seven cases in this paper, those where it is possible from the given data to obtain the absolute number of the eosinophil cells, we get the following results:

Case 29..............3·5 % eos.    14,000 per mm.[3]
"   30..............3·9 %  "      8,000    "
"   31..............3·4 %  "     11,000    "

The figure given by Zappert as a high normal value is 250. In these cases there is an average number of 11,000, that is 50 times as great. The observations then of Müller and Rieder themselves suffice fully to confirm Ehrlich's statement.

The absolute number of eosinophil cells depends naturally to a certain extent on the relative proportion of white to red corpuscles, and the greater the relative number of leucocytes, the greater should be the number of eosinophils. Zappert, for instance, found the following figures in his cases:

| Proportion of white to red corpuscles. | Absolute number of eosinophils. |
|---|---|
| 1 : 24 | 3,000—4,560 |
| 1 : 18 | 3,300 |
| 1 : 15 | 7,000 |
| 1 : 13 | 8,700 |
| 1 : 11 | 6,000 |
| 1 : 7·6 | 8,300 |
| 1 : 7·0 | 7,600 |
| 1 : 7·0 | 29,000 |
| 1 : 5·0 | 14,000 |
| 1 : 3·8 | 34,000. |

Apart from the approximate parallelism between the two rows of figures, this abstract shews that the minimal value—3,000 eosinophils with a proportion of white to red of 1 : 24—still amounts to 15 times the normal. The maximal figure found by Zappert of 30,000 is moreover by no means to be considered extreme. Cases of leukæmia are not infrequent in which we find 100,000 eosinophils per mm.³ and over.

From these figures it must be admitted that the absolute increase of the eosinophil cells in medullary leukæmia is not "alleged" (v. Limbeck) but on the contrary is very real and considerable.

That the absolute and relative number of eosinophil cells may markedly sink in certain complications of leukæmia, constitutes no exception to the law that the eosinophil cells are increased in myelogenic leukæmia. In this connexion the self-evident principle must be observed, that only analogous conditions are comparable. The standard of comparison for a leukæmic patient suffering from severe sepsis is not the blood of a healthy person with normal numerical proportions, but that of a patient similarly attacked by a severe sepsis. Now we know that in sepsis the number of eosinophil cells is enormously diminished, so that Zappert, in five cases of this nature, was unable to recognise any eosinophils in the blood. In contrast to this stands a case of myelogenic leukæmia described by Rieder and Müller, complicated by a severe and lethally ending suppurative process. In consequence of the acute neutrophil leucocytosis brought about by the septic infection, the number of eosinophils sank rapidly from 3·5 % to 0·43 % (4 hours before death). The absolute number of eosinophil cells however in this terminal stage still amounted to 1400—1500 per mm.³, and was therefore, in comparison with an uncomplicated sepsis, very much raised. Writers should not have disputed the importance of the eosinophil cells for the

diagnosis of leukæmia from cases like these; on the
contrary they should have seen in them a decisive confirmation of the constancy of the absolute increase of the
eosinophils in leukæmic blood.

At the time when Ehrlich formulated his proposition
on the diagnostic importance of the eosinophil cells in
leukæmia, the simple eosinophil leucocytosis (see p. 148),
first discovered later by the investigation of asthma etc.,
was unknown. For no confusion can arise between leukæmia, and conditions accompanied by eosinophilia, as
they can be distinguished on clinical grounds alone. The
blood moreover provides ample means for a differential
diagnosis: (1) the total increase of the white cells in this
case seldom reaches degrees that remind one of leukæmia;
(2) the eosinophil cells are exclusively polynuclear;
(3) mast cells and neutrophil myelocytes are almost
entirely absent.

In favour of the diagnostic value of the absolute
increase of the eosinophil cells are those cases too, where
with a blood condition closely recalling leukæmia, the
absence of eosinophil cells excludes the diagnosis of that
disease. In a case of carcinoma of the bone-marrow,
described by Epstein, with an anæmic constitution of
the blood (nearly always present it may be mentioned
in leukæmia), there was found a marked increase of the
white blood corpuscles, numerous neutrophil myelocytes
and nucleated red corpuscles. Anyone holding, as Müller
and Rieder do, that the number of eosinophil cells need
not be considered in the diagnosis, must in this case have
diagnosed myelogenic leukæmia. This however was according to Ehrlich's system impossible owing to the complete absence of eosinophil cells.

From all these observations it follows that an absolute

increase of eosinophil cells is indispensable for the diagnosis of leukæmia.

4. The absolute increase of the mast cells. The mast cells are always increased in myelogenic leukæmia. They may be counted in leukæmic blood with the aid of the triacid or eosine-methylene blue stain. As shewn by the former they appear as polynuclear cells free from granules, since their granulation takes on no dye of the triacid mixture.

In all cases of myelogenic leukæmia the increase of mast cells is absolute and considerable. Generally they are equally or half as numerous as the eosinophils, occasionally they may exceed the latter in number. Hence it follows that the mast cells undergo an increase in number relatively greater than the eosinophil cells, for they normally amount only to some $0.28\,^o/_o$. They are perhaps of greater diagnostic value than the eosinophils, because up to the present time we know of no other condition (in contradistinction to eosinophil leucocytosis) in which a marked increase of the mast cells occurs.

5. Atypical forms of the white corpuscles. Amongst these are to be mentioned: (a) dwarf forms of the polynuclear neutrophils and of the eosinophil elements respectively. As a rule they resemble normal polynuclear cells on a small scale. (b) Dwarf forms of the mononuclear neutrophil and eosinophil leucocytes, which correspond to the pseudo-lymphocytes described elsewhere (see p. 78). The importance of these dwarf forms for leukæmia is as yet insufficiently explained; and it is difficult to decide whether they are already small forms on reaching the blood-stream, or whether they are there produced by division of a large cell. (c) Cells with

12—2

mitoses. Formerly particular weight was laid on the observation of mitoses, for they were regarded as evidence that the increase of white blood corpuscles was brought about in the circulating blood itself, an assumption specially supported by Löwit.

A large number of authors (H. F. Müller, Wertheim, Rieder) have demonstrated mitoses, particularly of the myelocytes, in the circulating blood in leukæmia. No diagnostic importance of any kind can however be ascribed to them. They are found in all cases only in very small numbers. Thus Müller says that he generally must look through many thousands of white cells before meeting one mitosis. Only in one case did he find the figures of nuclear division somewhat more abundant, where there was one mitosis only to several hundreds of leucocytes.

These really negative observations shew that the mitoses play a completely negligeable part in the increase of the cells in the blood itself. For the diagnosis of leukæmia they are valueless.

6.   Nucleated red corpuscles form a constant constituent of leukæmic blood. In different cases their number is very varying ; in one case they occur extremely sparingly, in another every field contains very many. The normoblastic type is found most frequently, but side by side with it, megaloblasts and forms transitional between the two are occasionally found. Mitoses within the red blood discs have been described by different authors, but possess no theoretic or clinical importance. The appearance of erythroblasts in leukæmia may be either a specific phenomenon, or merely the expression of an anæmia accompanying the leukæmia. We are inclined to the first supposition, since the occurrence in such

numbers of nucleated red cells is hardly ever observed in other anæmias of the same severity.

So much for the characteristics of leukæmic blood, upon which the diagnosis of the disease is made. We must add that although in any case of medullary leukæmia each particular factor described is to be recognised, yet the manner of its appearance, its numerical relation to the others and to the total blood varies extremely. Apart from the degree of increase of the leucocytes, no one case is the same as another with regard to the other anomalies. In one case the blood bears a large-celled, mononuclear neutrophil character; in another the increase of the eosinophil cells predominates; in a third the nucleated red blood corpuscles preponderate; in a fourth we see a flooding of the blood with mast cells. And hence results a multiplicity of combinations, and each single case has its own individual features[1].

It is of special importance to study the changes due to certain inter-current diseases in the blood picture of medullary leukæmia. This point has recently been the object of detailed investigation, in particular by A. Fraenkel, Lichtheim and others[2]. According to these authors, under the influence of febrile diseases the total number of leucocytes may be enormously decreased. The blood moreover is altered, so that the myelæmic characteristics become less marked, and the polynuclear neutrophil elements largely preponderate. The latter may attain

[1] Ehrlich was once able to recognise, by balancing the different forms of cells, the blood preparations after the loss of their labels from some ten cases of leukæmia.

[2] Literature given by A. Fraenkel.

the percentage numbers of common leucocytosis up to 90 % and over.

We will here mention a few rare cases, demanding special attention, shewing the alterations leukæmic blood may undergo, and occasionally presenting almost insuperable difficulties in diagnosis. We find but a single case of this kind mentioned in the literature. Zappert reported a patient, who in February, 1892, had shewn the typical signs of myelogenic leukæmia. Amongst others the relation of white to red cells was found to be 1 : 4·92, and 1400 eosinophil cells per mm.³ (3·4 %) were counted. At the end of September of the same year the patient was brought in a miserable condition to the hospital, where she soon died with gradually failing strength. During this period of observation the proportion of white to red was 1 : 1·5; the percentage of eosinophils, 0·43; the mononuclears, most of which had no neutrophil granulation, amounted to 70 % of the leucocytes. Zappert expressly mentions that these mononuclear cells were in no way similar to the lymphocytes in general appearance. At the autopsy Zappert found the bone-marrow studded with non-granulated mononuclear cells, and the eosinophil cells were much more scanty than is usually the case in leukæmic bone-marrow. Blachstein, under Ehrlich's direction, investigated a second case of this kind. This patient had also been the subject of exact clinical investigations for some time on account of a myelogenic leukæmia. During the time he was last in hospital the blood could only be examined a day before the fatal termination, the direct consequence of a septic complication. With a markedly leukæmic constitution of the blood there were found 62 % polynuclear cells, 17·5 % mononuclear about the size of the ordinary myelocyte,

0·75 % eosinophil cells, nucleated red blood corpuscles in moderate amount. The preponderance of polynuclear and the small number of eosinophil cells is readily explainable from the septic infection; on the other hand the absence of granules in the mononuclear cells is most surprising.

These two observations can only be interpreted by assuming a loss, in certain terminal stages, on the part of the organism, of its power of forming neutrophil substances. Similar conditions occur in non-leukæmic conditions; for example in a striking case of posthæmorrhagic anæmia described by Ehrlich. It is of great importance to direct attention to these cases, which up to the present have been practically disregarded—for ignorance of their occurrence may easily give rise to gross errors concerning the nature and origin of the mononuclear cells, and to the manufacture of a lienal form of leukæmia.

Finally we have to discuss the important question, how **the origin of myelæmic blood** is to be explained. According to our conceptions two possibilities come under consideration. Either we have to deal with a passive inflow of bone-marrow elements, or with an active emigration from the bone-marrow into the circulation. This important and difficult question is certainly not fully ripe for discussion. The most weighty objection to be raised against an active emigration of the bone-marrow cells is derived from the behaviour of the white blood corpuscles on the warm microscopic stage. These investigations have been performed by a number of authors of whom may be mentioned Biesiadecki, Neumann, Hayem, Löwit, Mayet, Gilbert, and particularly H. F. Müller on the ground of his summary of this subject. Concerning the behaviour of the forms of cell here involved, all authors are agreed that under no conditions do the lymphocytes shew the smallest spontaneous movement; whilst the polynuclear neutrophil cells always exhibit vigorous contractility. With regard to the forms most characteristic of leukæmic blood the statements are partially contradictory. Some authors deny all spontaneous movement of these cells; but most of them report observations from which it follows that a certain power of spontaneous movement is not to be gainsaid. It will be admitted that in questions of this kind, negative results are weakened by positive data. Thus Jolly recently described similar observations as follows: "C'étaient des changements de forme sur place, lents et peu considérables, formations de bosselures à grands rayons, passage d'une forme arrondie à une forme ovulaire ou bilobée etc. Ces mouvements étaient visibles dans les observations I et IV et appartenaient surtout à des globules de grande taille." It is naturally impossible to decide if these minute movements suffice for a spontaneous locomotion. But one cannot exclude off-hand the supposition that they do. It is indeed supported by a further observation of Jolly on the mononuclear eosinophil cells of the marrow. Hitherto it was taken for established that these cells are completely devoid of spontaneous movement. Jolly however was recently able to examine a specimen from a case of typical leukæmia, in which nearly all the eosinophil cells shewed active movement. He says: "Ces globules granuleux actifs présentaient des mouvements de progression et des changements de forme caractéristiques et rapides; cependant je n'ai pas vu ces globules présenter de pseudopodes effilés; de

plus, leurs contours restaient presque toujours assez nette-
ment arrêtés. Ces particularités correspondent exactement
à la description, qu'a donnée depuis longtemps Max
Schultze des mouvements des cellules granuleuses du sang
normal." Examination of dry specimens from the same
case shewed, as Jolly expressly mentioned, that the blood
contained, as leukæmic blood always does, polynuclear
and mononuclear eosinophil cells. In contrast then with
all earlier observations, Jolly has demonstrated an active
spontaneous movement of the mononuclear eosinophil
cells. The amœboid movement of the mononuclear cells
is so seldom seen, not because they lack this function, but
obviously from defects in the methods of investigation,
which as is manifest are rather rough and wholly unsuited
for delicate biological processes. There are many instances
in the literature of the failures of this method, even in
the case of cells with undisputed mobility. Thus Rieder
failed to observe any contractility in the majority of
polynuclear leucocytes in a case of malignant lymphoma,
whereas according to all other observations they possess
this property without exception.

We think then we must draw the conclusion that the
feeble mobility of the mononuclear cells, both eosinophilous
and polynuclear, is only apparent, and is owing to the
gross method of investigation. In reality they doubtless
have mobility sufficient for emigration.

A further, but much less weighty objection to the
view that myelogenic leukæmia is an active leucocytosis
is, that pus artificially produced in leukæmic patients has
nearly always the histological constitution of normal pus.
But from our previous detailed remarks we should only
expect a myelæmic constitution of the pus, if the specific
morbid agent of leukæmia were present in a concentrated

form at the place of inflammation. Just as we saw in pemphigus, Neusser's eosinophilous suppuration occurred only in the specific pemphigus bullæ, but not in the foci of suppuration that were artificially produced. We know that the myelocytes are in no way positively influenced by the chemiotactic stimuli of ordinary infectious agents. On the contrary, it clearly follows from the above-mentioned observations on the transformation of leukæmic blood under the influence of infectious diseases, that the common bacterial poisons act in a negatively chemiotactic sense, both on the eosinophil and on the neutrophil mononuclear cells. Under these circumstances we should indeed expect that artificially produced suppuration in leukæmic patients would have, not a myelæmic, but a polynuclear neutrophil character.

It will be the task of further investigations to examine accurately inflammatory products, *e.g.* pleuritic exudations, in leukæmic patients, with the object of elucidating the question, whether under special conditions of disease all the leucocytes characteristic for leukæmia may not be able to wander from the blood. Thus in a case of pleurisy in a leukæmic patient, Ehrlich received the impression from the preparations that a "myeloid" emigration had in fact occurred, carrying all the elements in the blood into the exudation. This observation does not prove the point, for numerical estimation of the proportion of white to red blood corpuscles in the exudation was not made. And these estimations are necessary in order to prove indisputably the active emigration of the white blood corpuscles into the exudation, and to exclude their purely mechanical passage, *per rhexin*, from the blood-stream.

The hypothesis of the active origin of myelæmia is

considerably supported by a further train of argument. In leukæmia, besides the myelocytes, the polynuclear leucocytes are also enormously increased, and their active emigration is beyond doubt. And the view, that the mononuclear cells are washed into the blood, excludes that of a single mode of origin of the leukæmic blood condition; and commits us to a highly artificial explanation of its production.

The morphological changes of leukæmic blood under the influence of infectious diseases can only be explained from the standpoint of the emigration theory. For if the white blood corpuscles were mechanically carried out of the bone-marrow as a whole, it is incomprehensible that a bacterial infection should alter this process to a polynuclear leucocytosis. This change of character is easily explained on the other hand, as we have above shewn more in detail, by the assumption that ordinary bacterial poisons act positively chemiotactically only on the polynuclear neutrophil cells, but negatively on the other forms.

We explain the origin of leukæmic blood by the emigration into the blood under the influence of the specific leukæmic agent, not only of the formed polynuclear elements, but also of their mononuclear, eosinophil and neutrophil early stages; and to classify myelogenic leukæmia with the active leucocytoses.

## V.  DIMINUTION  OF  THE  WHITE  BLOOD
## CORPUSCLES  (LEUKOPENIA).

DIMINUTION of the white blood corpuscles plays—
comparatively with their increase—a very unimportant
*rôle* in clinical observations.  It occurs in but few
groups of diseases, and but seldom attains a marked
degree.  Koblanck has described a most marked fall in
the number of the colourless cells, in the following remarkable blood condition.  In a strong man, 25 years of
age, whose internal organs were found to be healthy,
short epileptiform attacks occurred, in one of which death
took place.  The autopsy gave no indication of the cause
of death.  Two examinations of the blood were made in
the course of the three days he was under observation.
In one of these, out of ten cover-glass preparations,
not a single white blood corpuscle was found, and
in the second only one example.

We have mentioned this case here, because it is
remarkable as an extreme leukopenia never before observed.  An explanation however is impossible owing to
the obscurity of the general clinical condition.

For the rest the conditions, under which a considerable

diminution of the leucocytes occurs, are very well-known.
We distinguish two chief groups :

1. Leukopenia from destruction of a portion of
the white blood corpuscles (Löwit);

2. Leukopenia from deficient inflow of white
corpuscles:

α. in infectious diseases from negative chemiotaxis;

β. in anæmia etc. from defective action of the
bone-marrow.

We have entered more fully into the leukopenia
experimentally produced by Löwit, in the chapter on
leucocytosis. We there explained, that according to
present views, we have to deal, not with an actual
destruction of the white elements, but merely with an
altered distribution within the blood-stream.

Amongst the infectious diseases where an hypoleucocytosis occurs, typhoid fever must first be mentioned. The
diminution is chiefly at the expense of the polynuclear
cells. Uncomplicated measles too, generally runs its course
with a marked leukopenia, specially distinct during the
breaking out and at the height of the exanthem. These
cases of infectious leukopenia are to be explained, not
by a destruction of white corpuscles, but rather by a
diminished inflow, brought about by the circulation of
substances negatively chemiotactic for the polynuclear
elements.

Leukopenia has still another meaning in certain cases
of severe anæmia, where it indicates a highly unfavourable
prognosis. Ehrlich has described (*Charité Annalen* 1888)
a case of posthæmorrhagic anæmia ending fatally, where
an extreme diminution of the leucocytes occurred. Exact
figures shewed that the greater proportion (80 %) of white

blood corpuscles consisted of lymphocytes, whilst the polynuclears amounted to 14°/₀ (instead of 70—72°/₀ normally).
Eosinophil cells and nucleated red blood corpuscles were
entirely absent. Ehrlich explained these phenomena by
a deficient activity of the bone-marrow, which found
expression in the insufficient formation of red and white
blood corpuscles. As the anatomical basis of this deficient
activity, he conjectured that in this case the fatty marrow
of the big long bones could not have been changed to
blood forming red marrow, as is the rule in severe
anæmias. In two cases the autopsy fully confirmed this
diagnosis made during life.

## The blood platelets.—The hæmoconiæ.

The **blood-platelets** were first described by Hayem,
later by Bizzozero, as a third formed element of normal
blood. They are roundish or oval discs free from hæmoglobin. They are extremely unstable under mechanical,
thermal, and chemical influences. Their size amounts to
some $3\mu$. Specially characteristic is their tendency, the
result of their extraordinary stickiness, to run together
into largish clumps, " grape clusters." This circumstance
greatly facilitates the distinction of the blood platelets
from the other formed elements, but renders their
enumeration most difficult. The apparatus usually used
for counting the blood corpuscles is, for this reason,
deceptive; for the platelets rapidly cling to its walls
and remain there. All early authors (*e.g.* Bizzozero)
endeavoured to obviate this error by some particular
diluting fluid; but a number of these elements still

remained fastened to the walls of the capillary tube of the mixing apparatus.

Recently Brodie and Russell have recommended a new mixture in which the platelets remain quite isolated, and are stained at the same time. They allow the drop of blood as it comes from the puncture to enter a drop of the fluid, and then estimate the relative proportion of red blood corpuscles to platelets[1]. The prescription for their solution is as follows:

Dahlia-glycerin,
$2^0/_0$ solution of common salt...equal parts.

Another method, used by the majority of more recent authors, is the relative enumeration of blood platelets in the stain dry specimen. Ehrlich found that the blood platelets were picked out by their deep red colour, corresponding to the amount of alkali they contain, in preparations treated by the iodine eosine method (see p. 46). Rabl's new method is much more complicated and in no way more serviceable, depending on a stain with iron hæmatoxylin recommended by E. Haidenhain for demonstration of the centrosomes. A process of Rosin's, not yet published, is more convenient. It consists in fixing the dry preparation for 20 minutes in osmic acid vapour, and staining in a concentrated watery solution of methylene blue.

---

With regard to the significance of the blood platelets, most authors, of whom we should before all

---

[1] The physiological figures found by Brodie and Russell with the aid of this method exceed considerably those of earlier authors. They found a proportion of platelets to erythrocytes of 1 : 85 or an absolute number of about 635,000 per mm.[3]

mention Hayem, Bizzozero, Laker, assume justifiably that they are preformed in the living blood. The view opposed to this, advocated more particularly by Löwit, that these forms first arise in the blood after it has left the vessels, we may describe on the grounds of our own extensive observations as inaccurate.

The blood platelets, on the grounds of their small size and complete lack of nuclear substance, are generally regarded as not analogous to real cells. Whether they represent intravital precipitation of substances of the plasma, or whether they are budded off from the cells, cannot at the present be decided with certainty, though many facts seem to support the latter assumption. That they contain glycogen (see p. 45), marks them as descendants of the blood cells. Moreover, appearances are often met with in dry preparations that arouse the suspicion that the platelets arise from the red blood corpuscles (Koeppe). Arnold has further observed processes of budding in the red blood corpuscles not only extravascularly but also intravascularly in the mesentery of young guinea-pigs, and has seen the elements that were cut off change into forms free from hæmoglobin.

Our knowledge too of the physiological function of the blood platelets still needs much amplification. The original view of Hayem, who regards the blood platelets as early stages of the red blood discs, and for this reason calls them " hæmatoblasts," is, according to the judgment of most hæmatologists, untenable.

Nearly all more recent papers, on the other hand (cp. Löwit's compilation), recognise the close connection of the blood platelets with coagulation, first observed by Bizzozero. Whether the substance of the platelets directly yields the material for fibrin formation, as Bizzozero holds, or whether according to the observations on thrombus production of Eberth and Schimmelbusch they play but a subordinate part, is not yet decided. To enter here into the chemical side of this complicated problem, would lead us much too far, and we will only refer to a few clinical observations which illustrate the relations between the clotting power of the blood and the number of platelets it contains.

Marked increase of the blood platelets occurs in chlorosis (Muir) and in post-hæmorrhagic anæmia (Hayem). In both conditions there is a decided increase in the clotting power of the blood. In contrast, is the important observation of Denys, who found in two cases of purpura, where as is well-known the clotting power of the blood is always much lowered or may even be entirely destroyed, only one morphological blood change, a very marked diminution of the blood platelets. Ehrlich likewise had occasion to examine a similar case, in which the blood platelets were entirely absent.

---

H. F. Müller has described a fourth formed constituent of the blood, and given it the name of "haemoconiae" or "blood atoms," "blood dust." It is found in the plasma of the blood as very small granule- or coccæ-like colourless corpuscles, highly refractile, with a very active molecular movement, which keep their shape under observation for a very long time without any special precautions. According to Müller these bodies are not blackened by osmic acid, and probably contain no fat; they seem to have no connection with fibrin formation, as they always

M. 13

lie outside the fibrin network. Müller found them in
every normal blood, in varying numbers however; much
increased in a case of Morbus Addisonii; diminished in
hunger and cachexias.

More detailed observations are necessary to determine
the chemical nature of these forms. Experiments in this
direction by extraction with ether, or by the use of fat
staining substances, alkanna, Soudan dye, and comparative
investigations on lipæmic blood should be successful.

# LITERATURE[1].

**Altmann.** Über die Elementarorganismen und ihre Beziehungen zu den Zellen. *Leipzig*, 1 Aufl. 1890. 2 Aufl. 1894.

**Arnold.** Zur Morphologie und Biologie des Knochenmarks. *Virchow's Archiv*, Bd. 140.

—— Über die Herkunft der Blutplättchen. *Centralbl. f. allg. Pathologie und path. Anat.* Bd. 8, 1897.

**Askanazy.** Über einen interessanten Blutbefund bei rapid letal verlaufender Anæmie. *Zeitschr. f. klin. Med.* 1893, Bd. 23.

—— Über Bothriocephalus-Anæmie, und die prognostische Bedeutung der Megaloblasten in anæmischem Blut. *Zeitschr. f. klin. Med.* 1895, Bd. 27.

**Barker.** On the presence of iron in the granules of the eosinophil leucocytes. *Johns Hopkins Hosp. Bull.* no. 42, 1894.

**Bäumer.** Beiträge zur Histologie der Urticaria simplex und pigmentosa, mit besonderer Berücksichtigung der Bedeutung der Mastzellen für die Pathogenese der Urticaria pigmentosa. *Inaugural Dissertation. Berlin*, 1895.

**Beck.** Über Quecksilber-Exantheme. *Charité Ann.* Bd. 20.

**v. Beck.** Subcutane Milzruptur, Milzexstirpation, Heilung. *Münch. Med. Woch.* 1897, no. 47.

**Benario.** Noch einmal die Leucocytenschatten Klein's. *Deutsche Med. Woch.* 1894, no. 27.

---

[1] Owing to the enormous extent of hæmatological literature, we have been able to refer only to more recent publications. We have, however, indicated several papers, in which bibliographies of particular parts of the subject are to be found.

**Biernacki.** Untersuchungen über die chemische Beschaffenheit bei pathologischen, insbesondere bei anæmischen Zuständen. *Zeitschr. f. klin. Med.* 1894, vol. XXIV. (References to literature.)

**Bizzozero.** Über die Bildung der roten Blutkörperchen. *Virchow's Archiv*, 1884, vol. XCV.

—— Über einen neuen Formbestandtheil des Blutes, und dessen Rolle bei der Thrombose und der Blutgerinnung. *Virchow's Archiv*, 1882, vol. XC.

**Bleibtreu, L.** Kritisches über den Hæmatokrit. *Berl. klin. Woch.* 1893, nos. 30, 31.

**Bleibtreu, M. und L.** Eine Methode zur Bestimmung des Volums der körperlichen Elemente im Blut. *Pflüger's Archiv*, 1892, vol. LI.

**Blex-Hedin.** *Skandinavisches Archiv f. Path.* 1890 (quoted by Limbeck).

**Brodie and Russell.** The enumeration of blood-platelets. *Journ. of Physiology*, 1897, nos. 4 and 5.

**Brown, T. R.** *Johns Hopkins Hosp. Bulletin*, 1897.

**Buchner.** Untersuchungen über die bacterienfeindlichen Wirkungen des Blutes und Blutserums. *Arch. f. Hygiene*, vol. X, 1890.

**Bücklers.** Über den Zusammenhang der Vermehrung der eosinophilen Zellen im Blute mit dem Vorkommen der Charcot'schen Krystalle in den Fæces bei Wurmkranken. *Münch. Med. Woch.* nos. 2 and 3.

**Calleja.** Distribución y Significación de las Células cebadas de Ehrlich. *Rivista trimestr. micrográfica*, vol. I. 1896.

**Canon.** Über eosinophilen Zellen und Mastzellen im Blut Gesunder und Kranker. *Deutsche Med. Woch.* 1892, no. 10.

**Cohnheim.** Vorlesungen über allgemeine Pathologie. I. and II. *Berlin*, 1877.

**Cohnstein und Zuntz.** Untersuchungen über den Flüssigkeitsaustausch zwischen Blut und Geweben unter verschiedenen physiologischen und pathologischen Bedingungen. *Pflüger's Archiv*, 1888, vol. XLII.

**Crédé.** Über die Exstirpation der kranken Milz an Menschen. *Langenbech's Archiv*, 1883, vol. XXXVIII. (Literature.)

**Czerny.** Zur Kenntniss der glycogenen und amyloiden Entartung. *Arch. f. exp. Path. und Pharm.* 1893, vol. XXXI.

**Denys.** Un nouveau cas de Purpura avec diminution considérable des plaquettes. Revue: *La Cellule*, vol. v. pt. 1.

**Dieballa.** Über den Einfluss des Hæmoglobingehaltes und der Zahl der Blutkörperchen auf das specifische Gewicht des Blutes bei Anæmischen. *Deutsche Arch. f. klin. Med.* 1896, vol. LVII.

**Dock.** Zur Morphologie des leukæmischen Blutes. *Moscow Internat. Congress,* 1897.

**Dunin.** Über anæmische Zustände. *Leipzig,* 1895. *Volkmann's Sammlung klin. Vortrüge.* N.F. 135.

**Egger.** Über die Untersuchung der Blutkörperchen beim Aufenthalt im Hochgebirge. *Correspondenzbl. f. Schweizer Ärzte,* 1892, vol. XXXII. *Congress f. innere Med.* 1893, vol. XII.

**Ehrlich.** Farbenanalytische Untersuchungen zur Histologie und Klinik des Blutes. *Berlin,* 1891.

—— Beiträge zur Ätiologie und Histologie pleuritischer Exsudate. *Charité Ann.* 1880, vol. 7.

—— Zur Kenntniss des acuten Milztumors. *Charité Ann.* 1882, vol. IX.

—— Über schwere anæmische Zustände. *XI. Congress f. inn. Med.* 1892.

—— De- und Regeneration roter Blutscheiben. *Verhandl. d. Gesellsch. d. Charité Ärzte,* June 10 and Dec. 9, 1880.

—— **und Frerichs.** Über das Vorkommen von Glycogen im diabetischen und im normalen Organismus. *Zeitschr. f. klin. Med.* 1883, vol. 7.

**Einhorn.** Über das Verhalten der Lymphocyten zu den weissen Blutkörperchen. *Inaugural Dissertation. Berlin,* 1884.

**Elze.** Das Wesen der Rhachitis und Scrophulose und deren Bekämpfung. *Berlin,* 1897.

**Engel, C. S.** Hæmatologischer Beitrag zur Prognose der Diphtherie. *Verhandl. d. Vereins f. inn. Med. zu Berlin,* 1896, 1897.

—— Über verschiedene Formen der Leucocytose bei Kindern. *XV. Congr. f. inn. Med.* 1897.

**Epstein, J.** Blutbefunde bei metastatischer Carcinose des Knochen-marks. *Zeitschr. f. klin. Med.* 1896, vol. xxx.

**Eykmann.** Blutuntersuchungen in den Tropen. *Virchow's Archiv*, vol. cxxvi.

**Fano.** Quoted by **v. Limbeck.**

**Fischer, A.** Untersuchungen über den Bau der Cyanophyceen und Bacterien. *Jena*, 1897.

**Fraenkel, A.** Über acute Leukæmie. *Deutsche Med. Woch.* 1895, nos. 39—43.

—— **und Benda, C.** Klinische Mittheilungen über acute Leuk-æmie. *XV. Congr. f. inn. Med.* 1897.

**Frerichs.** Über den plötzlichen Tod und über das Coma bei Diabetes. *Zeitschr. f. klin. Med.* 1883, vol. vi.

**Gabbi.** Die Blutveränderungen nach Exstirpation der Milz, in Beziehung zur hæmolytischen Function der Milz. *Ziegler's Beiträge zur path. Anat.* vol. xix. pt. 3.

**Gabritschewsky.** Klinisch-hæmatologische Notizen. *Arch. f. exp. Path. u. Pharm.* 1891, vol. xxviii.

—— Mikroscopische Untersuchungen über Glycogenreaction im Blut. *Arch. f. exp. Path. u. Pharm.* 1891, vol. xxviii.

**Gärtner, C.** Über eine Verbesserung des Hæmokrit. *Berl. klin. Woch.* 1892, no. 36.

**Glogner.** Über das specifische Gewicht des Blutes des in den Tropen lebenden Europæers. *Virchow's Archiv*, vol. cxxvi.

**Goldberger und Weiss, F.** Die Jodreaction im Blut und ihre diagnostische Verwertung in der Chirugie. *Wiener klin. Woch.* 1897.

**Goldmann.** Beitrag zu der Lehre von dem "malignen Lymphom." *Centralbl. f. allgem. Path. u. path. Anat.* 1892, vol. iii.

**Goldscheider und Jakob.** Über die Variationen der Leucocytose (Literature). *Zeitschr. f. klin. Med.* vol. xxv. 1894.

**Gollasch.** Zur Kenntniss des asthmatischen Sputums. *Fortschritte d. Med.* 1889, vol. vii.

**Grawitz, E.** Über die Einwirkung des Höhenklimas auf die Zusammensetzung des Blutes. *Berl. klin. Woch.* 1895, Nos. 33, 34.

**Grawitz, E.** Klinische Pathologie des Blutes. *Berlin*, 1896.

—— Über Blutbefunde bei Behandlung mit dem Koch'schen Mittel. *Charité Ann.* 1891.

—— Klinisch-experimentelle Blutuntersuchungen. *Zeitschr. f. klin. Med.* 1892, vols. XXI. XXII.

**Gulland.** On the Granular Leucocytes. *Journ. of Physiol.* 1896, vol. XIX.

**Hahn, M.** Über die Beziehungen der Leucocyten zur bactericiden Wirkung des Blutes. *Archiv f. Hygiene,* 1895, vol. XXV.

**Hammerschlag.** Über das Verhalten des specifischen Gewichtes des Blutes in Krankheiten. *Centralbl. f. klin. Med.* 1891, no. 44.

—— Über Hydræmie. *Zeitschr. f. klin. Med.* 1892, vol. XXI.

—— Über Blutbefunde bei Chlorose. *Wiener Med. Presse,* 1894, no. 27.

**Hankin, E. H.** Über den Ursprung und das Vorkommen von Alexinen im Organismus. *Centralbl. f. Bakt. u. Parasitenkunde,* 1892, vol. XII.

**Hardy, W. B.** Wandering cells and bacilli. *Journ. of Physiol.* 1898.

—— Blood Corpuscles of Crustacea. *Journ. of Physiol.* 1892.

**Hartmann et Vaquez.** Les modifications du sang après la splénectomie. *Compt. rend. de la Société de Biologie.* Xth Series, vol. IV. 1897.

**Hayem.** Du sang. *Paris,* 1889.

—— Du caillot non rétractile. Suppression de la formation du sérum sanguin dans quelques états pathologiques. *Acad. des Sciences,* Nov. 1896. (Sem. médic.)

—— Des globules rouges à noyau dans le sang de l'adulte. *Arch. de Phys. norm. et path.* IIIrd Series, vol. I. 1883.

**Herz, Max.** Blutkrankheiten. *Virchow's Archiv,* vol. CXXXIII.

**Hirschfeld, H.** Beiträge zur vergleichenden Morphologie der Leucocyten. *Inaug. Dissert. Berlin,* 1897.

**Hoppe-Seyler.** Verbesserte Methode der colorimetrischen Bestimmung des Blutfarbstoffgehaltes im Blut und in anderen Flüssigkeiten. *Zeitschr. f. phys. Chemie,* vol. XVI.

**Howell.** The life-history of the formed elements of the blood. (Quoted by H. F. Müller.)

**Israel, O. und Leyden.** Demonstrationen in der Berliner medicinischen Gesellschaft. *Berl. klin. Woch.* 1890, no. 40.

**Israel und Pappenheim.** Über die Entkernung der Säugethiererythroblasten. *Virchow's Archiv,* vol. CXLIII.

**Jadassohn.** Demonstration von eosinophilen Zellen in Lupus und in anderen Geweben. *Verhandl. d. deutschen dermatolog. Gesellsch.* II. and III. Congress. (Quoted by H. F. Müller, Asthma bronchiale).

**v. Jaksch.** Über die prognostische Bedeutung der bei croupöser Pneumonie auftretenden Leucocytose. *Centralbl. f. klin. Med.* 1892, no. 5.

**Janowski, W.** Zur Morphologie des Eiters verschiedenen Ursprungs. *Arch. f. Path. u. Pharm.* 1895, vol. XXXVI.

**v. Jaruntowski und Schröder, E.** Über Blutveränderungen im Gebirge. *Münch. Med. Woch.* 1894, no. 48.

**Jenner.** A new preparation for rapidly fixing and staining blood. *Lancet,* 1899.

**Jolly, M. J.** Sur les mouvements amiboïdes des globules blancs du sang dans la Leucémie. *Compt. rend. de la Soc. de Biolog.* X. Series, vol. 5, 1898.

**Jones, Wharton.** *Philosophical Transactions,* 1846, vol. I.

**Kanter.** Über das Vorkommen von eosinophilen Zellen in malignem Lymphom und bei einigen anderen Lymphdrüsenerkrankungen. *Inaug. Dissert. Breslau,* 1893.

**Kanthack and Hardy.** The Morphology and Distribution of the wandering cells of Mammalia. *Journ. of Physiol.* 1894.

—— On the Characters and Behaviour of the Wandering Cells of the Frog, especially in relation to Micro-organisms. *Phil. Trans.* 1894.

**Kikodse.** Die pathologische Anatomie des Blutes bei der croupösen Pneumonie. *Inaug. Dissert.* (Russian). Reviewed in *Centralbl. f. allg. Path. u. path. Anat.* 1891, no. 3.

**Klebs.** Cp. *XI. Congr. f. inn. Med.* Discussion.

**Knoll.** Über die Blutkörperchen bei wirbellosen Thieren. *Sitzungsber. d. kais. Akademie d. Wissensch. in Wien.* Mathematisch-naturwissenschaftl. Cl. 1893, vol. CII. Pt 6.

**Koblanck.** Zur Kenntniss des Verhaltens der Blutkörperchen bei Anæmie, unter besonderer Berücksichtigung der Leukæmie. *Inaug. Dissert. Berlin,* 1889.

**Kœppe.** Über Blutuntersuchungen im Gebirge. *Congr. f. inn. Med.* 1893, vol. XII.

—— Über Blutuntersuchungen in Reiboldsgrün. *Münch. Med. Woch.* 1895.

—— Über den Quellungsgrad der roten Blutscheiben durch äquimoleculare Salzlösungen, und über den osmotischen Druck des Blutplasmas. *Arch. f. Anat. u. Phys.* Phys. Abt. 1895.

**Kündig.** Über die Veränderungen des Blutes im Hochgebirge bei Gesunden und Lungenkranken. *Correspondenzbl. f. Schweiz. Ärtze,* 1897, 1 and 2.

**Laache.** Die Anæmie. *Christiania,* 1883.

**Labadie-Lagrave.** Traité des maladies du sang. *Paris,* 1893.

**Laker.** Über eine neue klinische Blutuntersuchungs-methode. (Specifische Resistenz der roten Blutkörperchen.) *Wiener med. Presse,* 1890, no. 35.

—— Die Blutscheiben sind constante Formelemente des normal circulierenden Säugethierblutes. *Virchow's Archiv,* 1889, vol. CXVI.

**Landois, L.** Lehrbuch der Physiologie des Menschen. *Wien u. Leipzig,* 1887.

**Lazarus, A.** Blutbefund bei perniciöser Anæmie. *Verhandl. d. Vereins f. inn. Med. Deutsche Med. Woch.* 1896, no. 23.

**Leredde et Perrin.** Anatomie pathologique de la Dermatose de Dühring. *Ann. de Dermat. et Syphilograph.* IIIrd Series, VI.

**Lewy, Benno.** Über das Vorkommen der Charcot-Leyden'schen Krystalle in Nasentumoren. *Berl. klin. Woch.* 1891, nos. 33 and 34.

**Leyden, E.** Über eosinophile Zellen aus dem Sputum von Bronchialasthma. *Deutsche Med. Woch.* 1891, no 38.

**Lichtheim.** Leukæmie mit complicierender tuberculöser Infection. *Verein f. wissenschaftl. Heilkunde zu Königsberg,* Feb. 1897.

**v. Limbeck.** Grundriss einer klinischen Pathologie des Blutes. 2nd Ed. *Jena,* 1896.

—— Über die durch Gallenstauung bewirkten Veränderungen des Blutes. *Centralbl. f. inn. Med.* 1896, no. 33.

**Litten.** Über einige Veränderungen roter Blutkörperchen. *Berl. klin. Woch.* 1877, no. 1.

**Löwit.** Die Blutplättchen, ihre anatomische und chemische Bedeutung. Reviewed in Lubarsch-Ostertag's *Ergebn. d. allgem. Path. Wiesbaden,* 1897. (Literature.)

—— Protozoennachweis im Blute und in den Organen leukæmischer Individuen. *Centralbl. f. Bakt.* 1898, vol. XXIII.

**Lœwy, A.** Über Veränderungen des Blutes durch thermische Einflüsse. *Berl. klin. Woch.* 1896, no. 4.

—— **und Richter, P. F.** Über den Einfluss von Fieber und Leucocytose auf den Verlauf von Infectionskrankheiten. *Deutsche Med. Woch.* 1895, no. 15.

—— —— Zur Biologie der Leucocyten. *Virchow's Archiv,* 1898, vol. CLI.

**Lyonnet.** De la densité du sang. *Paris,* 1892.

**Maragliano.** Beitrag zur Pathologie des Blutes. *XI. Congress f. inn. Med.* 1892.

**Maxon.** Untersuchungen über den Wasser- und den Eiweissgehalt beim kranken Menschen. *Deutsches Archiv f. klin. Med.* 1894, vol. LII'.

**Mayer, Karl Hermann.** Die Fehlerquellen der Hæmometer-Untersuchung (v. Fleischl). *Deutsches Archiv f. klin. Med.* vol. LVII. (Abundant references.)

**Mayer, S.** Über die Wirkung der Farbstoffe Violett B. und Neutralroth. *Sitzungsb. d. deutschen naturwissensch.-med. Vereins f. Böhmen. Lotos,* 1896, no. 2.

**Mendel, K.** Ein Fall von myxœdematösem Cretinismus. *Berl. klin. Woch.* 1896, no. 45.

**Menicanti.** Über das specifische Gewicht des Blutes und dessen Beziehungen zum Hæmoglobingehalt. *Deutsches Archiv f. klin. Med.* 1892, vol. L.

**Mercier.** Des modifications de nombre et de volume que subissent les erythrocytes sous l'influence de l'altitude. *Arch. de Physiologie.* Vth Series, VI. 1894.

**Meunier.** De la leucocytose dans la coqueluche. *Compt. rend. de la Soc. de Biologie.* Xth Series, V. 1898.

**Michaelis, L.** Beiträge zur Kenntniss der Milch-secretion. *Arch. f. mikr. Anat. u. Entwicklungsgeschichte,* vol. LI. 1898.

—— Die vitale Färbung, eine Darstellungsmethode der Zellgranula. *Arch. f. mikrosc. Anat. u. Entwicklungsgeschichte,* 1900.

**Miescher.** Über die Beziehungen zwischen Meereshöhe und Beschaffenheit des Blutes. *Correspbl. d. Schweiz. Ärzte,* 1892, 23.

**Mosler.** Die Pathologie und Therapie der Leukæmie. *Berlin,* 1872.

**Muir, R.** Contribution to the physiology and pathology of the blood. *Journ. of Anat. and Phys.* vol. XXV. 1891.

**Müller, H. F.** Die Morphologie des leukæmischen Blutes und ihre Beziehungen zur Lehre von der Leukæmie (Summary). *Centralbl. f. allg. Path. u. path. Anat.* vol. V. nos. 13 and 14.

—— Zur Leukæmie-Frage. *Deutsches Arch. f. klin. Med.* vol. XLVIII.

—— Über die atypische Blutbildung bei der progressiven perniciösen Anæmie. *Deutsches Arch. f. klin. Med.* 1893, vol. LI.

—— Zur Lehre vom Asthma bronchiale. *Centralbl. f. allg. Path. u. path. Anat.* 1893, vol. IV.

—— **und Rieder.** Über Vorkommen und klinische Bedeutung der eosinophilen Zelle im circulierenden Blut des Menschen. *Deutsches Arch. f. klin. Med.* vol. XLVIII.

—— —— Über einen bisher nicht beachteten Formbestandtheil des Blutes. *Centralbl. f. allg. Path. u. path. Anat.* 1896.

**Neumann, E.** Über Blutregeneration und Blutbildung. *Zeitschr. f. klin. Med.* 1881, vol. III.

—— Farblose Blut- und Eiterzellen. *Berl. klin. Woch.* 1878, no. 41.

**Neumann, E.** Ein neuer Fall von Leukæmie mit Erkrankung des Knochenmarks. *Arch. d. Heilkunde*, 1872, vol. XIII.

**Neusser.** Über einen besonderen Blutbefund bei uratischer Diathese. *Wien. klin. Woch.* 1894, no. 39.

—— Klinisch-hæmatologische Mittheilungen (Pemphigus). *Wien. klin. Woch.* 1892, nos. 3 and 4.

**v. Noorden.** Untersuchungen über schwere Anæmie. *Charite Ann.* 1889, vol. XVI.

—— Beiträge zur Pathologie des Asthma bronchiale. *Zeitschr. f. klin. Med.* vol. XX.

**Nothnagel.** Lymphadenia ossium. *Internat. klin. Rundschau,* 1891. (Quoted by **Epstein**.)

**Pappenheim.** Die Bildung der roten Blutscheiben. *Inaug. Dissert. Berlin,* 1895. (Ample references.)

—— Über Entwicklung und Ausbildung der Erythroblasten. *Deutsche Med. Woch.* 1897, vol. XLVIII.

**Pée.** Untersuchungen über Leucocytose. *Inaug. Dissert. Berlin,* 1890.

**Peiper.** Zur Symptomatologie der tierischen Parasiten. *Deutsche Med. Woch.* 1897, no. 48.

**Perles.** Beobachtungen über perniciösen Anæmie. *Berl. klin. Woch.* 1893, no. 40.

**Pfeiffer, Th.** Über die Bleibtreu'sche Methode zur Bestimmung des Volums der körperlichen Elemente im Blut und die Anwendbarkeit derselben auf das Blut gesunder und kranker (insbesondere fiebernder) Menschen. *Centralbl. f. inn. Med.* 1895, no. 4.

**Prowazek.** Vitalfärbungen mit Neutralroth an Protozoën. *Zeitschr. f. wissenschaftl. Zoolog.* 1897.

**Prus.** Eine neue Form der Zellenartung. Secretorische fuchsinophile Degeneration. *Centralbl. f. allg. Path. u. path. Anat.* 1895, vol. VI.

**Przesmycki.** Über die intravitale Färbung des Kernes und des Protoplasmas. *Biolog. Centralbl.* vol. XVII. nos. 9 and 10. (Extensive bibliography on nuclear staining.)

**Pugliese.** Über die physiologische Rolle der Riesenzellen. *Fortschr. d. Med.* 1897, vol. XV. no. 19.

**Quincke.** Weitere Beobachtungen über perniciöse Anæmie. *Deutsches Arch. f. klin. Med.* vol. xx.

—— Zur Physiologie und Pathologie des Blutes. *Deutsches Arch. f. klin. Med.* vol. xxiii.

—— Über Eisentherapie. *Volkmann's Sammlung klin. Vorträge.* N.F. 129.

**Rabl.** Über eine elective Färbung der Blutplättchen in Trockenpräparaten. *Wien. klin. Woch.* 1896, no. 46.

**Rählmann.** Über einige Beziehungen der Netzhautcirculation zu allgemeinen Störungen des Blutkreislaufes. *Virchow's Archiv,* vol. cii.

**Reinbach.** Über das Verhalten der Leucocyten bei malignen Tumoren. *Langenbech's Archiv,* 1893, vol. xlvi.

**Reinert.** Die Zählung der roten Blutkörperchen. *Leipzig,* 1891.

**Ribbert.** Beiträge zur Entzündung. *Virchow's Archiv,* 1897, vol. cl.

**Rieder.** Atlas der klinischen Mikroscopie des Blutes. *Leipzig,* 1893.

—— Beiträge zur Kenntniss der Leucocytose (Literature). *Leipzig,* 1892.

**Rindfleisch.** Über Knochenmark und Blutbildung. *Arch. f. mikr. Anat.* 1880.

—— Über den Fehler der Blutkörperchenbildung bei der perniciösen Anæmie. *Virchow's Archiv,* 1890, vol. cxxi.

**v. Roietzky.** Contributions à l'étude de la fonction hæmatopoïétique de moëlle osseuse. *Arch. des sciences biol. Pétersbourg,* 1877. T. V.

**Sadler.** Klinische Untersuchungen über die Zahl der corpusculären Elemente und den Hæmoglobingehalt des Blutes. (Quoted by **Türk.**) *Fortschr. d. Med.* 1892.

**Schauman.** Zur Kenntniss der sogenannten Bothriocephalus-Anæmie. *Berlin,* 1894.

—— **und Rosenquist.** Zur Frage über die Einwirkung des Höhenklimas auf die Blutbeschaffenheit (Prelim. Comm.). *Congr. f. inn. Med.* 1896, no. 22.

**Schiff.** Über das quantitative Verhalten der Blutkörperchen und des Hæmoglobins bei neugeborenen Kindern und Säuglingen unter normalen und pathologischen Verhältnissen. *Zeitschr. f. Heilkunde*, 1890, vol. ii.

**Schimmelbusch.** Die Blutplättchen und die Blutgerinnung. *Virchow's Archiv*, 1885, vol. ci.

**Schmaltz.** Die Untersuchung des specifischen Gewichtes des menschlichen Blutes. *Deutsch. Arch. f. klin. Med.* 1891, vol. xlvii.

—— Die Pathologie des Blutes und der Blutkrankheiten. *Leipzig,* 1896.

**Schmidt, A.** Demonstration mikroscopischer Präparate zur Pathologie des Asthma. *Congr. f. inn. Med.*

**Schultze, Max.** Ein heizbarer Objecttisch und seine Verwendung bei Untersuchung des Blutes. *Arch. f. mikr. Anat.* 1865, vol. i.

**Schultze, O.** Die vitale Methylenblaureaction der Zellgranula. *Anatom. Anzeiger,* 1887.

**Schumburg und Zuntz, N.** Zur Kenntniss der Einwirkungen des Hochgebirges auf den menschlichen Organismus. *Pflüger's Archiv,* 1896, vol. lxiii.

**Seige.** Über einen Fall von Ankylostomiasis. *Inaug. Dissert. Berlin,* 1892.

**Spilling.** See **Ehrlich,** Farbenanalytische Untersuchungen.

**Stiénon.** Recherches sur la leucocytose dans la Pneumonie aigue. *Bruxelles,* 1895.

—— De la leucocytose dans les maladies infectueuses. *Bruxelles,* 1896.

**Stierlin.** Blutkörperchenzählung und Hæmoglobinbestimmung bei Kindern. *Deutsches Arch. f. klin. Med.* 1889, vol. xlv.

**Stintzing und Gumprecht.** Wassergehalt und Trockensubstanz des Blutes beim gesunden und kranken Menschen. *Deutsches Arch. f. klin. Med.* 1894, vol. xliii.

**Tarchanoff, J. R.** Die Bestimmung der Blutmenge am lebenden Menschen. *Pflüger's Archiv,* vols. xxiii, xxiv.

**Teichmann.** Mikroscopische Beiträge zur Lehre von der Fett-resorption. *Inaug. Dissert. Breslau,* 1891.

**Thoma und Lyon.** Über die Methode der Blutzählung. *Virchow's Archiv,* vol. LXXXIV.

**Troje.** Über Leukæmie und Pseudoleukæmie. *Berl. klin. Woch.* 1892, no. 12.

**Tschistowitsch.** Sur la quantité des leucocytes du sang dans les pneumonies fibrineuses à issue mortelle. Review : *Centralbl. f. d. Med. Wissensch.* 1894, no. 39.

**Türk.** Klinische Untersuchungen über das Verhalten des Blutes bei acuten Infectionskrankheiten. *Wien u. Leipzig,* 1898.

**Unger.** Das Colostrum. *Virchow's Archiv,* vol. CLI. 1898.

**Unna.** Über mucinartige Bestandtheile der Neurofibrome und des Centralnervensystems. *Monatshefte f. prakt. Dermatologie,* 1894, vol. XVIII.

**Uskoff,** and the papers of his pupils. See *Archiv des sciences biologiques,* St Pétersbourg.

**Uthemann.** Zur Lehre von der Leukæmie. *Inaug. Dissert. Berlin,* 1888.

**Viault.** Sur l'augmentation considérable du nombre des globules rouges dans le sang chez des habitants des hauts-plateaux de l'Amérique du Sud. *Compt. rend. d. l'Acad. des Sciences,* III.

**Virchow.** Weisses Blut (Leukæmie). *Virchow's Archiv,* vol. I.

—— Cellular-Pathologie. 4th Ed. *Berlin,* 1871.

**Waldstein.** Beobachtungen an Leucocyten u. s. w. *Berl. klin. Woch.* 1895, no. 17.

**Weiss.** Hæmatologische Untersuchung. *Wien,* 1896.

—— Über den angeblichen Einfluss des Höhenklimas auf die Hæmoglobinbildung. *Zeitschr. f. phys. Chem.* 1896—1897, vol. XXII.

**Wendelstadt, H. und Bleibtreu, L.** Beitrag zur Kenntniss der quantitativen Zusammensetzung des Menschenblutes unter pathologischen Verhältnissen. *Zeitschr. f. klin. Med.* 1894, vol. XXV.

—— —— Bestimmung des Volumens und des Stickstoffgehaltes des einzelnen roten Blutkörperchens in Pferde- und Schweine-blut. *Pflüger's Archiv,* vol. LII.

**Westphal.** Über Mastzellen. *Inaug. Dissert. Berlin*, 1880. (Cp. **Ehrlich**, Farbenanalytische Untersuchungen.)

**Winternitz.** Weitere Untersuchungen über Veränderungen des Blutes unter thermischen Einwirkungen. *Wiener klin. Woch.* 1893, no. 47.

**Wolff, F. und Kœppe.** Über Blutuntersuchungen in Reiboldsgrün. *Münch. med. Woch.* 1893, no. 11.

**Wright.** Remarks on methods of increasing and diminishing the coagulability of the blood. *Brit. Med. Journal*, 1894.

**Zangemeister.** Ein Apparat für colorimetrische Messungen. *Zeitschr. f. Biologie*, 1896, vol. XXII.

**Zappert, J.** Über das Vorkommen der eosinophilen Zellen im anæmischen Blut. *Zeitschr. f. klin. Med.* vol. XXIII. (Literature.)

—— Neuerliche Beobachtungen über das Vorkommen des Ankylostomum duodenale bei den Bergleuten. *Wiener klin. Woch.* 1892, no. 24.

**Zenoni, C.** Über das Auftreten kernhaltiger roter Blutkörperchen im circulierenden Blut. *Virchow's Archiv*, 1895, vol. CXX.

**Zesas, G.** Beitrag zur Kenntniss der Blutveränderung bei entmilzten Menschen und Tieren. *Langenbech's Arch.* 1883, vol. XXVIII.

# INDEX.

Printed in the United States
By Bookmasters